OECD Health Policy Studies

Waiting Times for Health Services

NEXT IN LINE

OECD

BETTER POLICIES FOR BETTER LIVES

This work is published under the responsibility of the Secretary-General of the OECD. The opinions expressed and arguments employed herein do not necessarily reflect the official views of OECD member countries.

This document, as well as any data and map included herein, are without prejudice to the status of or sovereignty over any territory, to the delimitation of international frontiers and boundaries and to the name of any territory, city or area.

The statistical data for Israel are supplied by and under the responsibility of the relevant Israeli authorities. The use of such data by the OECD is without prejudice to the status of the Golan Heights, East Jerusalem and Israeli settlements in the West Bank under the terms of international law.

Please cite this publication as:
OECD (2020), *Waiting Times for Health Services: Next in Line*, OECD Health Policy Studies, OECD Publishing, Paris, *https://doi.org/10.1787/242e3c8c-en*.

ISBN 978-92-64-75437-9 (print)
ISBN 978-92-64-98904-7 (pdf)

OECD Health Policy Studies
ISSN 2074-3181 (print)
ISSN 2074-319X (online)

Foreword

Long waiting times for health services have been an important policy issue in most OECD countries for many years as they generate dissatisfaction for patients because the expected benefits of diagnoses and treatments are postponed, and the pain and discomfort remain while people wait. The current COVID-19 pandemic will likely increase waiting times for a range of non-urgent health services in many countries at least in the short-term as a result of treatment and elective surgery being rescheduled and postponed.

Governments in many countries took various measures before the COVID-19 outbreak to reduce waiting times, often supported by additional funding, with mixed success. Waiting times for elective treatment, which is usually the longest wait, stalled between 2010 and 2019 in many countries, and started to rise again in some others prior to the COVID-19 pandemic.

This report was prepared for the most part in 2019 before the COVID-19 crisis. It first reviews the importance of waiting times issues across OECD countries, based on responses to a policy questionnaire administered in 2019 and information gathered directly from citizens through population-based surveys. Second, it provides an overview of how waiting times differ across OECD countries up to 2019, focussing on waiting times for consultations with general practitioners (GPs), specialist consultations and elective treatments, based on survey data and the regular OECD data collection on waiting times for elective surgery. Third, it reviews evidence about the impact of waiting times on access to care and health outcomes for patients, using data on unmet medical care needs from the European Union Survey of Income and Living Conditions (EU-SILC) and a review of the literature from different countries. The fourth and main part of this report reviews a range of policy interventions that countries have used before the COVID-19 pandemic to tackle waiting times for different services, including elective surgery, primary care, cancer care and mental health services, with a focus on identifying successful policies.

The preparation of this report was led by Luigi Siciliani (University of York) and Gaetan Lafortune (OECD). Rie Fujisawa (OECD) and Sabine Vuik (OECD) provided useful data analysis and prepared the section on waiting times for cancer care and primary care, respectively. Emily Hewlett (OECD) drafted the section on waiting times for mental health services. Francesca Colombo (Head of the OECD Health Division) provided useful comments on different parts of this report. Lucy Hulett and Natalie Corry helped in preparing and finalising the manuscript.

The authors of the report thank officials from Health Ministries who provided valuable comments on an earlier draft during the OECD Health Committee meeting that was held in Paris on 11-12 December 2019. They are also grateful to all the officials from Health Ministries who responded to the policy and data questionnaire that was administered in 2019, which provided a large part of the information contained in this report.

Table of contents

FIGURES

TABLES

Follow OECD Publications on:

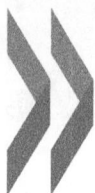

http://twitter.com/OECD_Pubs

http://www.facebook.com/OECDPublications

http://www.linkedin.com/groups/OECD-Publications-4645871

http://www.youtube.com/oecdilibrary

http://www.oecd.org/oecddirect/

Executive summary

The presence of waiting times in the health sector has been a long-standing challenge in many OECD countries, and the current COVID-19 pandemic will likely worsen waiting times for many non-urgent health services at least in the short-term. At the same time, waiting times are a reflection of the functioning of the health system as a whole and provide an opportunity for policy makers to trigger changes to improve the appropriateness, responsiveness and efficiency in health service delivery and to make health systems more people centred.

Waiting times for elective (non-urgent) treatment, which is usually the longest wait, have stalled over the past decade in many countries, and started to rise again in some others even before the COVID-19 outbreak. In response to the COVID-19 crisis, many countries have postponed elective surgery at least temporarily sometime during the first half of 2020 to free up a maximum amount of human resources and hospital beds to deal with the emergency. The postponement of these elective surgery will result in an immediate increase in waiting times for patients on the waiting lists and will result in a significant backlog of surgery that will likely take some time to be resolved after the crisis.

In normal circumstances, waiting times and waiting lists generally arise as the result of an imbalance between the demand for and the supply of health services. This can be for a consultation with a general practitioner or a specialist, or getting a diagnostic test or surgical or other elective treatments. Although some waiting times can improve the efficiency in the utilisation of resources by reducing idle capacity, when waiting times become long (e.g. above two or three months for elective treatments) more resources will need to be devoted by providers to manage waiting lists and prioritise patients and patient dissatisfaction will increase.

Several policies can be successfully implemented to reduce waiting times. Denmark, England and Finland succeeded in reducing waiting times for many elective health services and maintained these reductions over sustained periods, at least before the current COVID-19 crisis. The right policy mix for each country is likely to depend on the health system. However, successful approaches typically combine the specification of an appropriate maximum waiting time together with supply-side and demand-side interventions and a regular monitoring of progress.

All countries that want to address waiting times inevitably start by specifying a maximum waiting time, which requires a robust information system based on reliable data and definitions that capture the patient experience along the care pathway. There is no "one-size-fit-all" maximum waiting time. Countries have different maximum waits that reflect what can realistically be achieved given their starting point, the overall health spending, the additional resources they are willing to invest, and different institutional arrangements, payment systems and bottlenecks.

In some countries, maximum waiting times have been used as a target for providers and/or a guarantee for patients. Maximum waiting times have been used in England and Finland as targets with penalties for providers not meeting them. To meet the targets, providers need to implement demand and supply-side actions. Waiting time guarantees have been used in Denmark and Portugal and linked with patient choice policies, with patients being able to choose alternative health providers, including the private sector, if their waiting time approaches or exceeds the maximum.

On the supply side, only permanent and sustained increases in supply can lead to permanent reductions in waiting times. Lessons learned from past policies are that short-term interventions providing one-off additional funding do not have long-term effect on waiting times. Several countries (e.g. Australia, Canada, Estonia, Hungary, Ireland, the Netherlands, Poland and Slovenia) have allocated funding to increase the supply of services in some priority areas. Increasing the supply of services can be done in various ways. First, if there is slack in the system, then improving the management and efficiency in delivery (for example, through a better use of operating theatres) can be implemented at a relatively low cost. Increasing the productivity of providers is another option, for example by asking them to work additional sessions (and being adequately rewarded for it) or by introducing activity-based payment systems, though these are possible only if doctors and other members of health care teams have spare time and capacity to do more. Increasing the medical workforce is another option, if the productivity of the current workforce is already optimised, and if the physical and technical equipment (e.g. number of operating theatres) allows it, but this will be more expensive and will take more time before the effect can be felt.

However, even permanent increases in supply are not a guarantee of success. The main risk is that the additional supply is offset by an increase in demand, through an increase in referrals, tests and procedures, some of which may be inappropriate. For example, waiting times for some elective surgery in Canada and Australia have increased in recent years despite additional funding and surgical activities. Countries need to ensure that supply-side policies are linked to maximum waiting time enforcement to avoid disappointment. To ensure reductions in waiting times, a demand-side approach is also necessary to rationalise either GP referrals to specialists, or the propensity of specialists to add patients to a waiting list. In this respect, maximum waiting time targets (as used in England and Finland) can act as an indirect policy lever to ensure that when supply increases, providers do not offset these by increasing demand (through supply-induced demand or inappropriate referrals) but rather reduces the number of patients on the list, thereby translating into reduced waiting times.

Policy makers can also introduce several complementary and more direct approaches on the demand side to reduce waiting times for elective treatment (as in New Zealand). In the presence of large excess demand, clinical prioritisation tools that distinguish between patients with different health benefits and severity, can improve the referral process and the management of waiting lists. Prioritisation policies can also help to re-allocate waiting times by ensuring that patients with more severe conditions wait less than those with less severe conditions (as in Norway). Strengthening the referral systems from primary to secondary care, and improving the coordination between primary and secondary care, is another key policy in countries like Costa Rica, Finland and Poland, to ensure that resources are used efficiently and reduce waiting times.

OECD countries increasingly measure waiting times beyond elective treatment, including for primary care, cancer care and mental health services. Waiting times in primary care are less often considered a policy concern than for elective care, and only a few countries (such as Finland, Norway, and Spain) have implemented maximum waiting times to get an appointment with a general practitioner or other primary care providers. Policies to reduce waiting times in primary care often focus on increasing the supply of general practitioners, nurses and appointment slots. At the same time, more and more countries (such as Australia, Luxembourg and Estonia) have started to use new technologies to increase the supply of care (e.g. by offering teleconsultations) and to better manage demand (e.g. by allowing patients to more easily find doctors with availability and short waiting times).

Waiting times for cancer care are often shorter than for other types of care because of the urgency to get proper diagnosis and initiate treatment. In the majority of OECD countries, reducing waiting times for cancer care is considered an issue. More than half of OECD countries have developed waiting time strategies for cancer care covering both diagnosis and treatment, sometimes as part of national cancer control plans. Most countries set maximum waiting time targets and regularly evaluate their progress. Countries, such as Denmark, Ireland, Latvia, Poland, Slovenia and Spain, have also introduced fast track pathways for cancer patients, sometimes facilitated by additional dedicated funding and capacity. As for other elective treatment, increasing surgical activity rates for different types of cancer does not provide any guarantee that waiting times will fall if the demand increases. Countries, such as Finland, Greece, Japan, Luxembourg, the Netherlands, and Slovenia, have reorganised and streamlined cancer care delivery and improved coordination to achieve efficiency gains.

Waiting times policies for mental health services appear to be focused mainly on better meeting demand through increased service volumes or scope, rather than managing demand, possibly due to historical underfunding of mental health. Discussion of policies specifically tailored to reduce waiting times, or to improve the rate at which maximum wait time targets were met, was difficult to find. However, it appears that in some cases waiting time targets are part of a drive to increase overall access to mental health services, linked to a broader recognition that a significant treatment gap exists in the area of mental health. In some countries, such as Australia and England, new waiting time targets for mental health services have been introduced along with additional funding to increase service capacity, or even to introduce new service offers.

1 Waiting times remain an important policy issue in most OECD countries

Improving the experience and satisfaction of patients with the health care system is a key policy objective. Reducing the time that people have to wait to get access to health services can go a long way in improving patient experience, so that people don't feel that they are waiting too long to get proper diagnosis of their health problem and access to treatments to improve their health.

Waiting times can occur for a wide range of health services (Box 1.1). Regardless of the type of health care needed, waiting times are the result of the demand for health services being greater than the supply. This may be due either to capacity constraints or inefficiencies in referral processes and health service delivery, resulting in a queue and patients have to wait. In traditional markets, prices are used to ration goods and services and bring together demand and supply. In the health sector, due to public or private insurance, people face zero or low co-payments and there is therefore very limited reduction in demand due to prices. Instead, in publicly-funded systems, rationing for non-emergency treatment occurs through waiting times. In some health systems, when patients face longer waiting times, some patients may choose not to wait and opt for private treatment, provided they can afford to pay out of pocket or hold private health insurance. This might raise issues of equity in access.

Box 1.1. Different waiting times may occur for different types of health services

Several possible waiting times may arise along the patient journey as shown in Figure 1.1. For non-urgent care, patients will typically seek an appointment with a primary care physician (a general practitioner or GP) and wait from a few hours to several days. Following a GP visit, they may be referred to a specialist and wait days, weeks or months for an appointment. Patients may also wait for a diagnostic test, if required, such as an MRI and CT scan and/or for surgery or other treatment. Waiting for an elective surgical treatment is typically the longest, in the order of weeks, months or even years in some health systems.

Within elective care, certain treatments are more urgent than others if health is likely to deteriorate quickly without intervention, as for cancer and cardiac care. Patients with these health conditions tend to be prioritised over treatments for other conditions where health is less likely to deteriorate, such as for an elective hip replacement or cataract surgery.

Figure 1.1. Possible waiting times for different health services

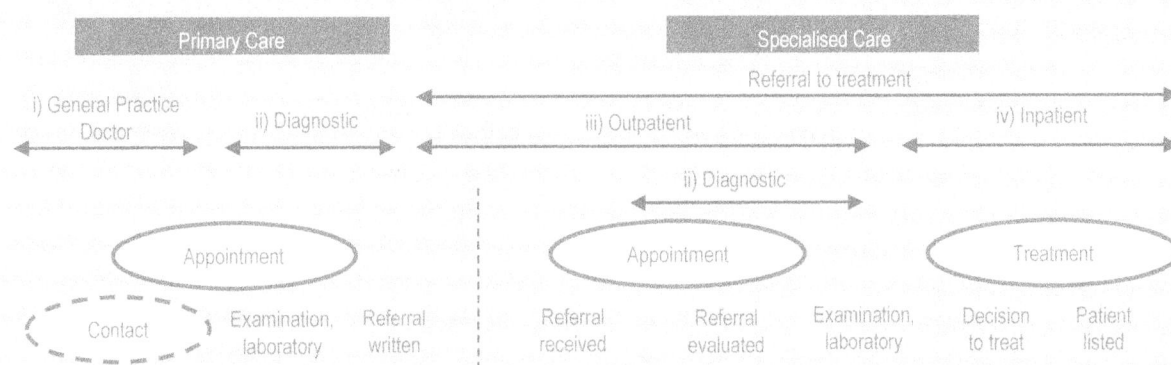

Source: Adapted from Siciliani, Borowitz and Moran (2013[1]), *Waiting Time Policies in the Health Sector: What Works?*, OECD Health Policy Studies, https://dx.doi.org/10.1787/9789264179080-en.

Waiting times for health services in publicly-funded systems aim to create equality between patients: patients with similar needs are supposed to wait their turn irrespective of their ability to pay or other non-clinical characteristics. Despite this rationale, several studies have found inequalities in waiting times by income or educational level even in publicly-funded health systems (Siciliani, 2015[2]). Beyond concerns about inequalities, another concern with rationing through waiting times is that the wait may worsen the health outcomes for patients. The available evidence shows that the effect on health outcomes depends on the duration of the wait, the health problem and the clinical prioritisation.

Although patients will seek health care in response to symptoms and illness, doctors have a significant role to play in determining how the demand for better health translates into a demand for health care or other treatments (e.g. pharmaceutical prescriptions). A large body of literature shows that there is unexplained variation in medical practice and overuse of diagnostic tests and procedures, which can be due to clinical uncertainty, clinical traditions and training, and supply-induced demand when activities are paid by fee for service (Wennberg, 2010[3]; OECD, 2014[4]; OECD, 2017[5]).

Responses to the OECD policy questionnaire administered for this project show that waiting times is considered to be either a high priority issue or at least a medium-high priority issue in most OECD countries (Figure 1.2). As expected, these include many countries with a national health system where all the population is covered for services mainly through tax revenues and where waiting times have often been a longstanding issue. However, it is also considered a growing priority issue in some countries that are based on social health insurance systems (such as Luxembourg and Slovak Republic). On the other hand, waiting times is not considered to be a significant policy issue in Germany, Korea, Japan, Switzerland and the United States. However, none of these countries report any statistics on waiting times except for Japan[1].

Figure 1.2. Waiting times are an important policy priority in many OECD countries, but not all

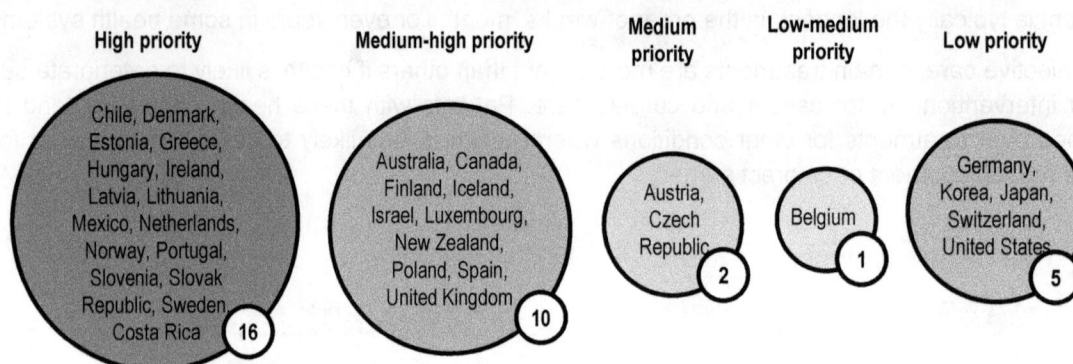

| High priority | Medium-high priority | Medium priority | Low-medium priority | Low priority |

Chile, Denmark, Estonia, Greece, Hungary, Ireland, Latvia, Lithuania, Mexico, Netherlands, Norway, Portugal, Slovenia, Slovak Republic, Sweden, Costa Rica — 16

Australia, Canada, Finland, Iceland, Israel, Luxembourg, New Zealand, Poland, Spain, United Kingdom — 10

Austria, Czech Republic — 2

Belgium — 1

Germany, Korea, Japan, Switzerland, United States — 5

Source: Based on responses from 34 countries to the OECD Waiting Times Policy Questionnaire (information is missing from three countries: France, Italy and Turkey).

In some countries, waiting times are considered to be an issue across a wide range of services, while in others waiting times are a significant issue only for some services (Figure 1.3). For example, in the Czech Republic and the Netherlands, waiting times are considered to be an issue mainly for elective treatments and mental health services.

In most countries, the main concern is about waiting times for elective treatments, followed by waiting times for specialist consultations and care. Nonetheless, in at least half of the countries, waiting times are an issue for other services, including primary care/GP consultations, hospital emergency department visits, access to diagnostic tests, as well as to more specific diagnostic and treatment in the area of cancer care, cardiac care and mental health services.

Figure 1.3. Waiting times are considered to be an issue across different types of health services

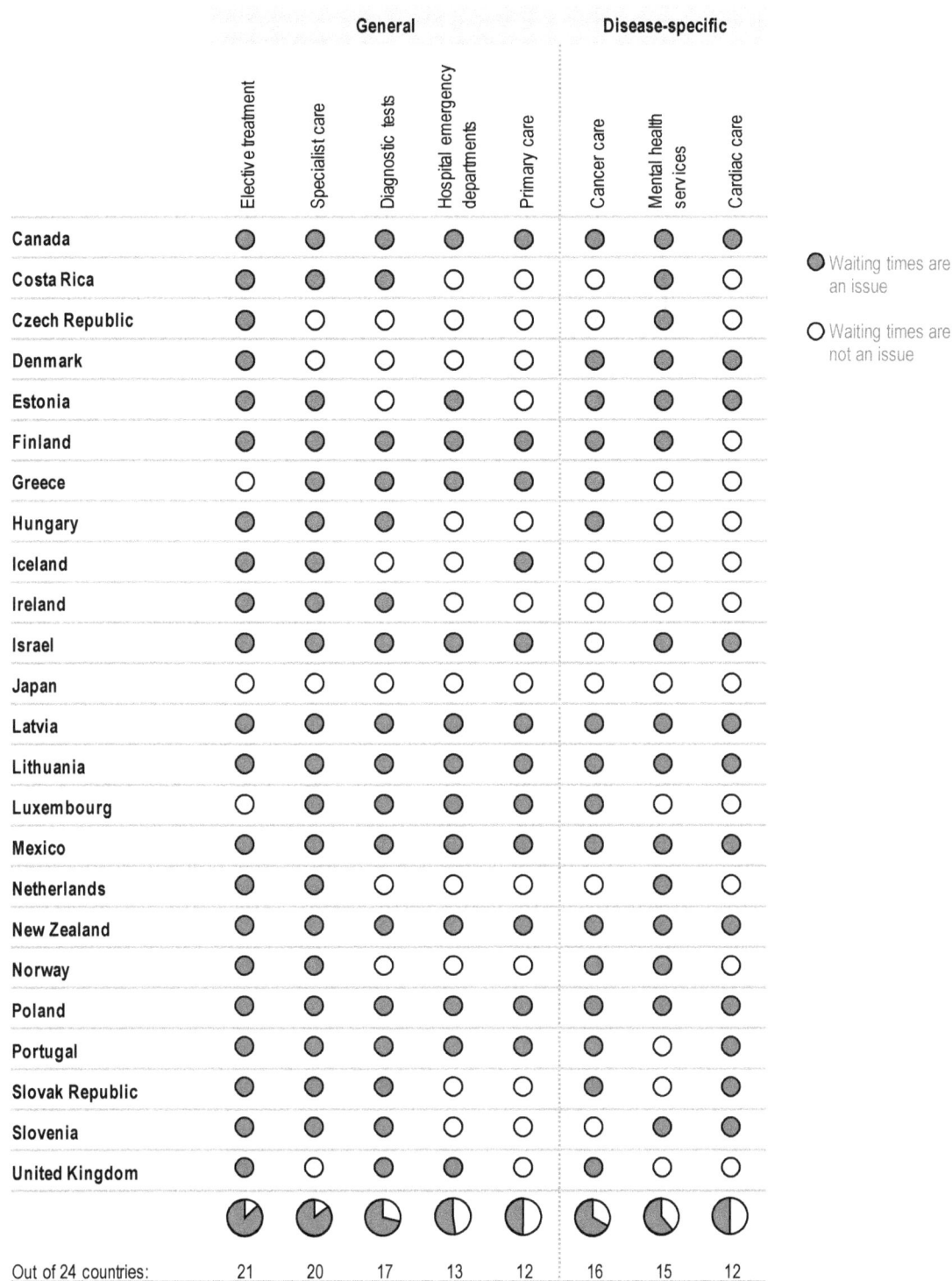

Legend: ● Waiting times are an issue ○ Waiting times are not an issue

	General					Disease-specific		
	Elective treatment	Specialist care	Diagnostic tests	Hospital emergency departments	Primary care	Cancer care	Mental health services	Cardiac care
Canada	●	●	●	●	●	●	●	●
Costa Rica	●	●	●	○	○	○	●	○
Czech Republic	●	○	○	○	○	○	●	○
Denmark	●	○	○	○	○	●	●	●
Estonia	●	●	○	●	○	●	●	●
Finland	●	●	●	●	●	●	●	○
Greece	○	●	●	●	●	●	○	○
Hungary	●	●	●	○	○	●	○	○
Iceland	●	●	○	○	●	○	○	○
Ireland	●	●	●	○	○	○	○	○
Israel	●	●	●	●	●	○	●	●
Japan	○	○	○	○	○	○	○	○
Latvia	●	●	●	●	●	●	●	●
Lithuania	●	●	●	●	●	●	●	●
Luxembourg	○	●	●	●	●	●	○	○
Mexico	●	●	●	●	●	●	●	●
Netherlands	●	●	○	○	○	○	●	○
New Zealand	●	●	●	●	●	●	●	●
Norway	●	●	○	○	○	●	●	○
Poland	●	●	●	●	●	●	●	●
Portugal	●	●	●	●	●	●	○	●
Slovak Republic	●	●	●	○	○	●	○	●
Slovenia	●	●	●	○	○	○	●	●
United Kingdom	●	○	●	●	○	●	○	○
Out of 24 countries:	21	20	17	13	12	16	15	12

Source: Based on responses from the OECD Waiting Times Policy Questionnaire 2019.

2 How long are waiting times across countries?

The definition and measurement of waiting times varies significantly across OECD countries, limiting the comparability of data. For non-emergency care, the measurement can use different start and end points. As shown in Figure 1.1 in Box 1.1, the waiting time can be recorded from the GP referral or following a specialist visit. It can end with a surgery or medical treatment, or with a specialist visit. Some health systems will measure what is sometimes referred to as the "outpatient" waiting time (from GP referral to specialist visit), others the "inpatient" waiting time (from a specialist decision to add the patient on the list to treatment), yet others measure the full referral-to-treatment waiting time (from GP referral to treatment), as is the case in Denmark, Norway and England.

For any health services, it is possible to measure and report the mean waiting time, the median waiting time or the waiting time at other percentiles of the distribution, and the number or proportion of patients waiting more than a threshold waiting time (for example 3, 6 or 12 months). The distribution of waiting times is generally skewed, with a small proportion of patients waiting a very long time. Hence, the mean waiting times can be substantially longer than the median.

Information on waiting times can be collected through administrative databases or surveys. One advantage of surveys is that they can often readily be used to measure any inequalities in waiting times across socio-economic groups, but one downside is that the data may be less reliable particularly if the sample size is small and may also become outdated if the surveys are not conducted regularly.

Annex A describes in more detail good practices in some countries in setting information systems to measure waiting times.

2.1. Waiting times for GP and specialist consultations vary more than two-fold across countries

According to the 2016 Commonwealth Fund International Health Policy Survey conducted in 11 OECD countries (Box 2.1), most people in 2016 were able get an answer to their medical concern from their regular doctor's office on the day when they contacted the office, although in some countries it was easier to get such a quick answer (Figure 2.1). The share of people reporting that they "sometimes, rarely or never get an answer from their regular doctor's office on the same day" was low in Switzerland (12%), Germany (13%) and the Netherlands (13%), but higher in Canada (33%) and the United States (28%). In most countries, this share did not change significantly between 2013 and 2016, although the survey results show progress in Australia and Switzerland, and suggest some deterioration in Sweden.

Box 2.1. The Commonwealth Fund International Health Policy Survey

Over the past 20 years, the Commonwealth Fund has coordinated the use of a household health survey across a number of OECD countries to collect a wide range of information, including on waiting times for GP consultations, specialist consultations and elective surgery. The number of OECD countries participating in this International Health Policy Survey has increased from five initially to eleven for the last wave in 2016 (Australia, Canada, France, Germany, the Netherlands, New Zealand, Norway, Sweden, Switzerland, United Kingdom and United States). While the sample size in some countries is fairly small, some countries have decided to increase the sample size to improve data reliability (e.g. there were over 5 000 respondents in Australia, over 4500 respondents in Canada and over 7 000 respondents in Sweden for the last wave in 2016).

Figure 2.1. The share of people who sometimes, rarely or never get an answer from their regular doctor's office on the same day varies by more than two-fold across countries

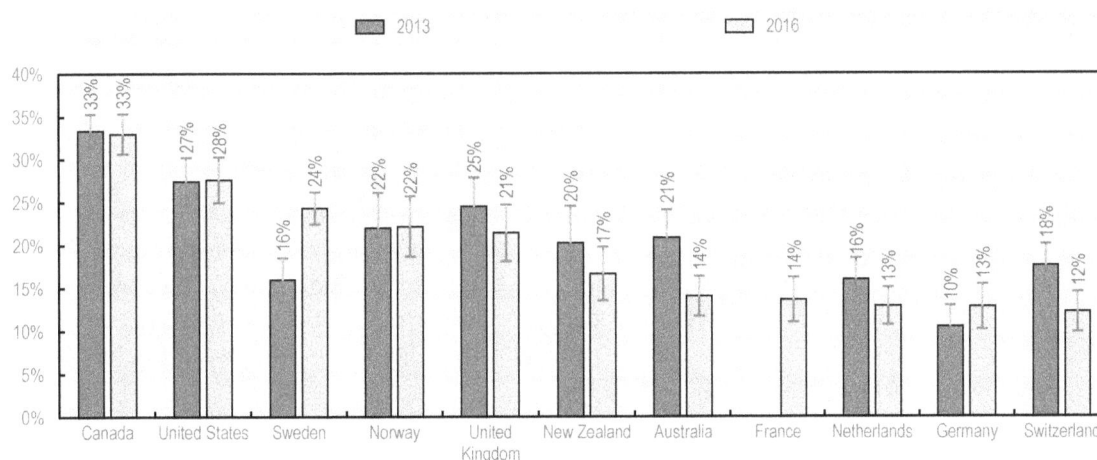

Note: 95% confidence intervals are shown by H.
Source: OECD calculations based on 2013 and 2016 Commonwealth Fund International Health Policy Surveys.

Turning to specialist care, waiting times for a specialist appointment also vary significantly across countries participating in the Commonwealth Fund survey (Figure 2.2). In 2016, the difference across countries was more than two-fold: over 60% of people waited one month or more for a specialist appointment in Canada and Norway, compared with about 25% only in Switzerland, Germany and the Netherlands. In many countries, waiting times for a specialist appointment has remained fairly stable between 2010 and 2016, although the survey results suggest that the situation has worsen in Norway, the United Kingdom and the United States.

Figure 2.2. The share of people waiting one month or more for a specialist appointment is two-times greater in some countries than in others

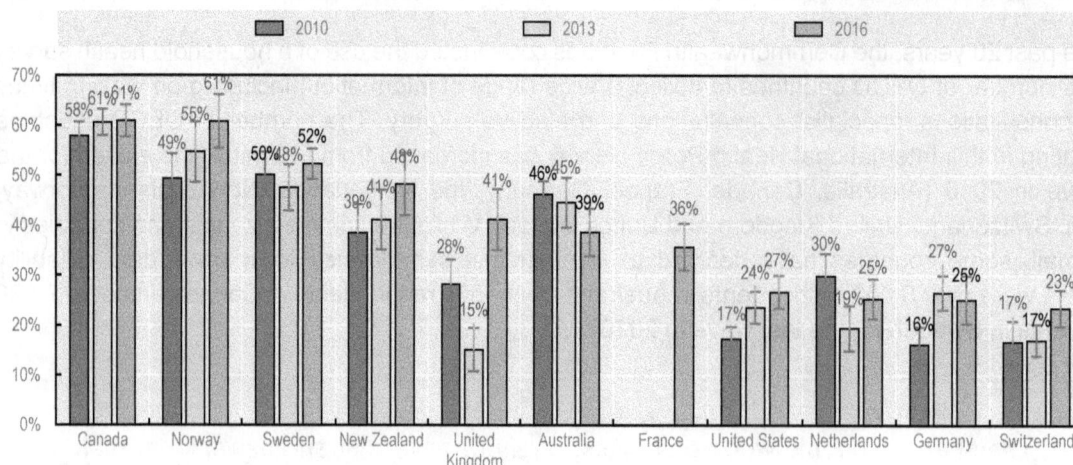

Note: 95% confidence intervals are shown by H.
Source: OECD calculations based on 2013 and 2016 Commonwealth Fund International Health Policy Surveys.

2.2. Waiting times for elective surgery is nearly ten-fold higher in some countries

Results from the regular OECD data collection on waiting times for common elective surgery show that they vary even more across the group of 17 OECD countries that report these data (which are based mainly on administrative sources). On average across these OECD countries, the median waiting times for more minor surgery like cataract operation was 95 days in 2018, and longer for more major surgery like hip replacement (110 days) and knee replacement (140 days). However, there are huge variations across countries. In general, waiting times for elective surgery in 2018 were the lowest in Denmark, the Netherlands, Italy and Hungary (where reducing waiting times for elective surgery is a key goal under the 2014-2020 Health Sector Strategy), while they were the highest in Estonia, Poland and Chile.

Looking at specific surgical procedures, Figure 2.3 shows that:

- The median waiting times for a cataract surgery varied from less than 40 days in Italy, Denmark and Hungary, to over 180 days (6 months) in Estonia and 250 days (over 8 months) in Poland.
- The median waiting times for a hip replacement was about 50 days or less in Denmark, Hungary, Italy and the Netherlands, compared with 240 days (about 8 months) or more in Estonia and Chile.
- The median waiting times for a knee replacement ranged from about 50 days or less in Italy, Denmark and the Netherlands, to 460 days (about 15 months) in Estonia and 840 days (about 28 months) in Chile.

Among the group of countries that have very long waiting times, the median waiting times for cataract surgery in Estonia decreased sharply between 2008 and 2013 (from over 300 days to 100 days), but then increased to reach more than 180 days in 2018. Recent trends in waiting times for hip replacement and knee replacement are even worse, with waiting times increasing greatly to levels exceeding those of ten years ago. In Chile, the median waiting times for hip replacement remained stable at around 240 days between 2013 and 2018. With regards to knee replacement, waiting times decreased from about 1 150 days (more than 3 years) in 2013 to 840 days (2 years and 4 months), but is still by far the longest. In Poland, the median waiting times fell sharply between 2013 and 2018 for cataract surgery and hip replacement, but still remain relatively high.

Among the group of countries that have relatively short waiting times now, Italy and the Netherlands have managed to keep waiting times for elective surgery relatively short in recent years (despite tight budgetary constraints in the case of Italy), while Denmark and Hungary have managed to reduce waiting times through a combination of policy actions (see Section 4).

Figure 2.3. Waiting times for common surgery vary from less than a month to over a year

Median waiting time from specialist assessment to treatment in days

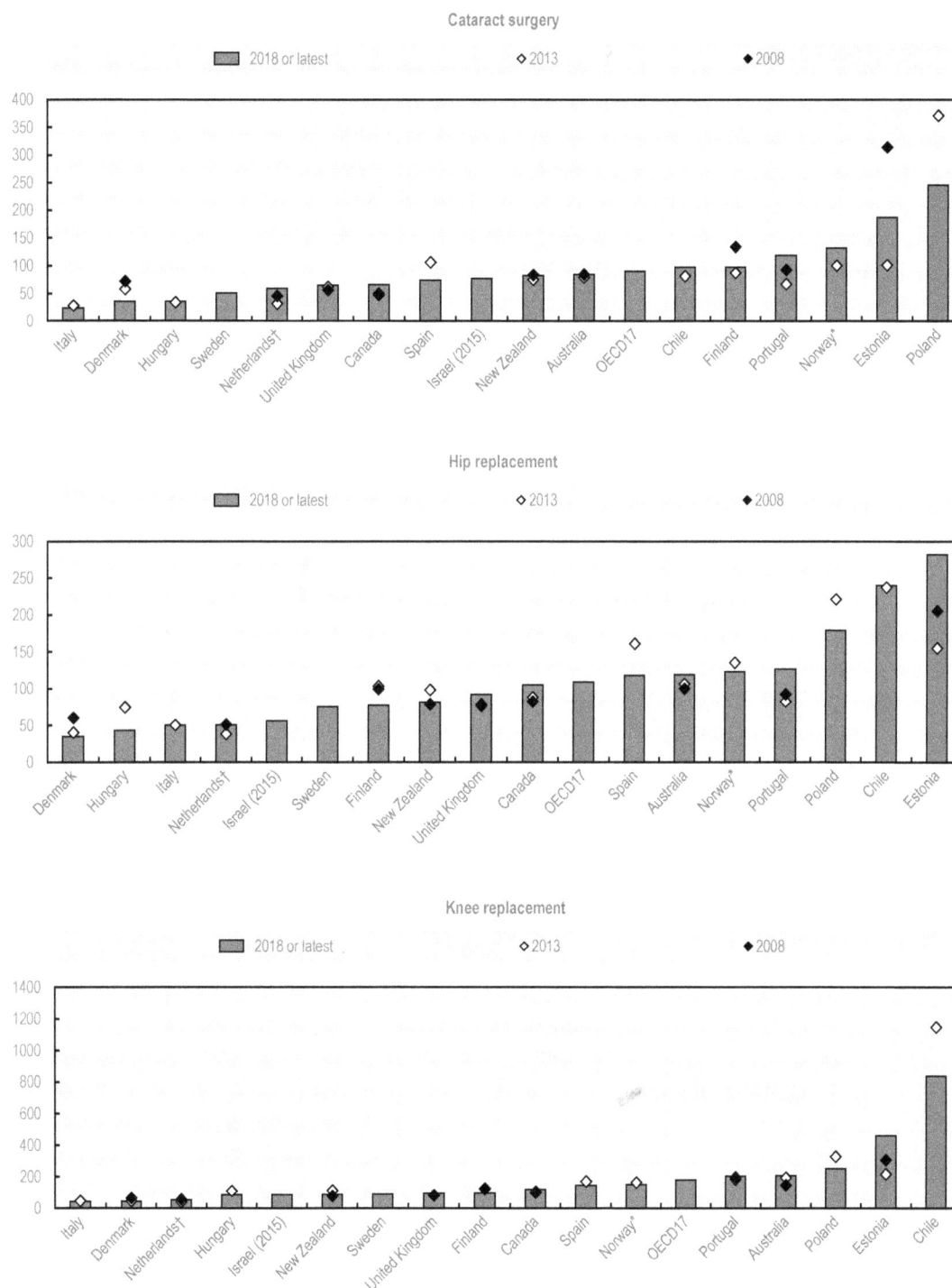

Note: † For the Netherlands, the data on waiting times is the mean number of days because the median is not available (resulting in an over-estimation compared with other countries). * For Norway, waiting times are over-estimated because they start from the date when a doctor refers a patient for specialist assessment up to the treatment (whereas in other countries they start only when a specialist has assessed the patient and decided to add the person on the waiting list for treatment).
Source: OECD Health Statistics.

In all countries, patients requiring more urgent treatments generally wait less than those whose health status is less likely to deteriorate while waiting. Prioritisation arises not only for people requiring the same treatment, but also across treatments (Gravelle and Siciliani, 2008[6]), as reflected for example by the fact that cancer patients wait significantly less than patients requiring a hip replacement. For instance, median waiting times for coronary bypass, hysterectomy and prostatectomy are generally shorter than for hip and knee replacement (Table 2.1).

Table 2.1. Waiting times are generally shorter for more urgent treatments

Median waiting times for selected elective surgery (days) OECD countries, 2018

	Cataract surgery	Hip replacement	Knee replacement	Hysterectomy	Prostatectomy	Coronary bypass	Coronary angioplasty
Australia	84	119	209	61	44	17	
Canada	66	105	122		40	6	
Chile	97	240	839	57	69	26	
Denmark	36	35	44	23	36	10	15
Estonia	187	282	461				
Finland	97	77	99	55	39	15	23
Hungary	36	43	85		10	22	
Israel	77	56	85	31	36	5	
Italy	24	50	42	33	36	9	11
New Zealand	82	81	89	80	66	62	38
Norway	132	123	152	118	105	62	43
Poland	246	179	253				27
Portugal	119	126	204	77	81	5	
Spain	74	118	147	55	75	37	35
Sweden	51	75	90	32	45	7	
United Kingdom	65	92	98	54	35	55	39
OECD average	**92**	**113**	**189**	**56**	**51**	**24**	**29**

Source: OECD Health Statistics.

When looking at the people who are still on the waiting lists and have not been treated yet, there are also large variations in the percentage of patients who have been waiting for over three months across the 12 countries that report these data. This proportion is lower in Hungary, New Zealand, Sweden and Spain for cataract surgery, and much higher in Slovenia, Estonia, Poland and Ireland (Figure 2.4).

In Slovenia, Poland and Estonia, the vast majority of patients (over 80%) on the waiting list for a cataract surgery or a hip or knee replacement has been waiting more than three months. This figure has been fairly stable in Poland and Estonia over the past 10 years. By contrast, in Sweden and New Zealand less than 25% of patients wait longer than three months, with this proportion coming down considerably in New Zealand since 2008.

Figure 2.4. The share of people waiting for over 3 months for common surgical procedures vary from less than 20% to over 80% across countries

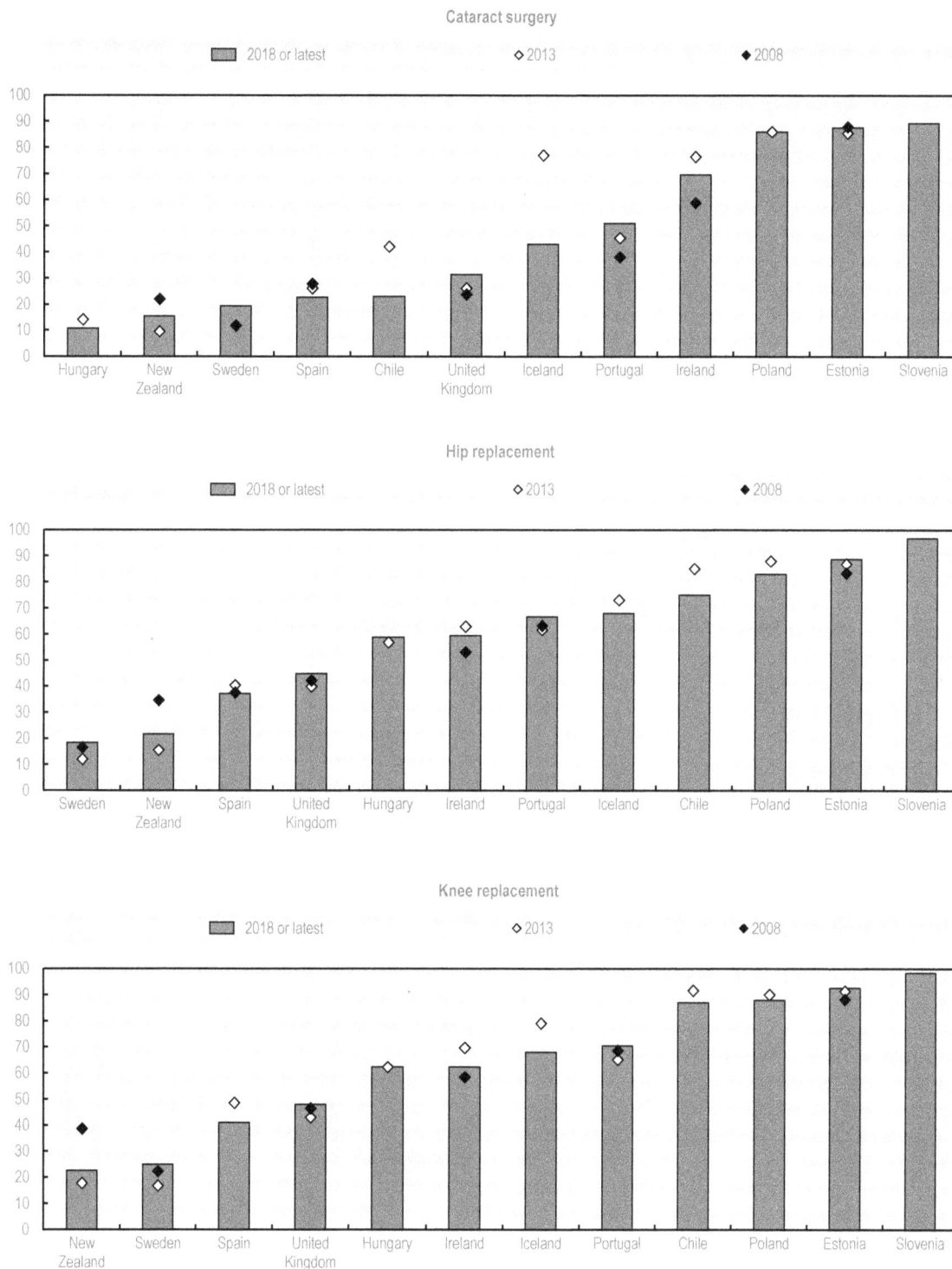

Cataract surgery

Hip replacement

Knee replacement

Source: OECD Health Statistics.

3 The impact of waiting times on access and health outcomes

A body of evidence shows that long waiting times can have negative effects on access to care and health outcomes for patients.

3.1. Waiting times can be an important source on unmet care needs in some countries

One possible consequence of waiting times is that they can prevent patients from receiving the care they need; and thus contribute to unmet needs. A European-wide survey (EU-SILC) shows that only a relatively small share of people report unmet care needs due to health system reasons in most countries. The share varies from less than 1% in Austria, the Czech Republic, Germany, Luxembourg, the Netherlands, Spain, Switzerland and Hungary, to over 10% in Estonia in 2018. It reached 5% to 10% of the population in Greece and Latvia (Figure 3.1). However, among people reporting unmet needs for health system reasons, waiting times is the main reason given in nearly 50% of cases on average across these European countries, followed by financial reasons. In Nordic countries, Slovenia, the United Kingdom, Estonia, Lithuania, Poland, the Slovak Republic and Ireland, most people who report unmet needs cite waiting times as the main reason (Figure 3.2).[2]

Figure 3.1. Unmet care needs related to the health system are generally low in Europe

% of population with unmet care needs due to the health system

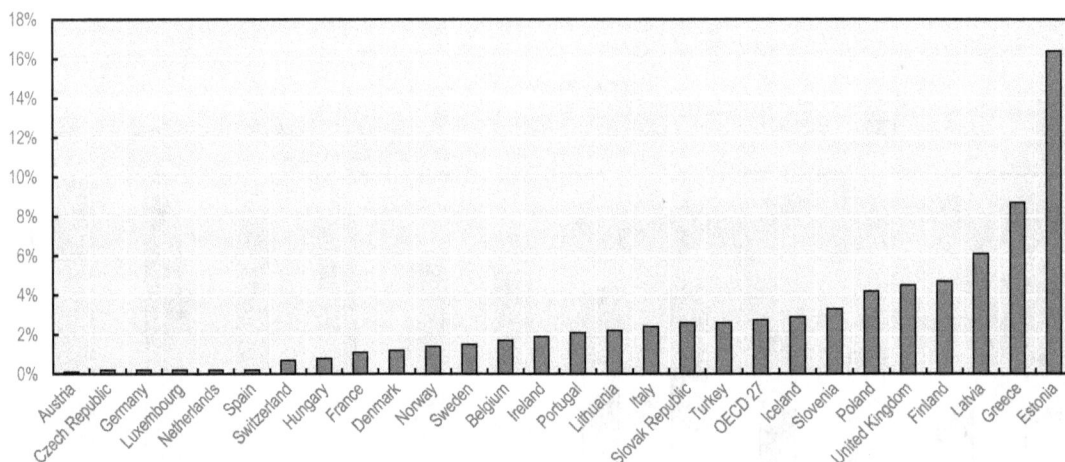

Source: European Union Statistics on Income and Living Conditions (EU-SILC) 2018 or latest year.

Figure 3.2. Waiting times are the main source of unmet care needs in several countries

% of health system unmet care needs due to waiting times and other reasons

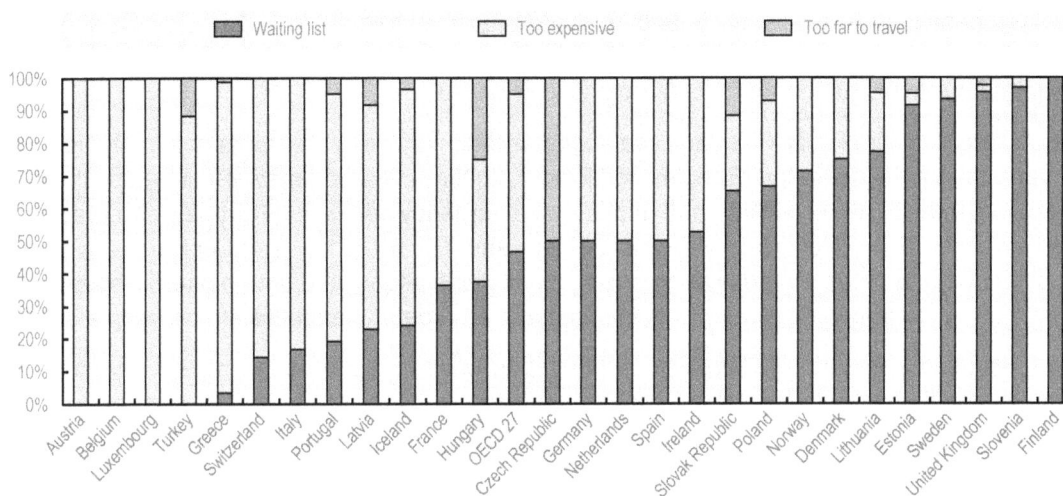

Source: European Union Statistics on Income and Living Conditions (EU-SILC) 2018 or latest year.

3.2. Waiting times may result in inequalities in access

While access to care is supposed to be based on need and not ability to pay in publicly-funded health systems, there is evidence of a certain degree of inequalities in waiting times by socio-economic status in many OECD countries.

Using large administrative data, inequalities have been found across several elective procedures, such as cataract surgery, hip and knee replacement, and coronary bypass, in many countries, including Australia (Johar et al., 2013[7]; Sharma, Siciliani and Harris, 2013[8]), England (Laudicella, Siciliani and Cookson, 2012[9]; Moscelli et al., 2018[10]), Norway (Monstad, Engesaeter and Espehaug, 2014[11]; Kaarboe and Carlsen, 2014[12]) and Sweden (Tinghög et al., 2014[13]; Smirthwaite et al., 2016[14]). Possible explanations for these inequalities include that individuals with higher socio-economic status live in neighbourhoods with higher availability of health care providers, translating into easier access. They may also exercise more patient choice in looking for providers with shorter waits, engage more actively with the system and exercise pressure when experiencing long delays, and have better social networks ("know someone").[3]

There is also evidence of socio-economic inequalities in waiting times from survey data. Using the Survey of Health, Ageing and Retirement in Europe (SHARE), Siciliani and Verzulli (2009[15]) provided evidence of socio-economic inequalities for specialist consultation in Spain, Italy and France, and for elective surgery in Denmark, the Netherlands and Sweden. Using survey data from Spain, Abásolo, Negrín-Hernández and Pinilla (2014[16]) found that people with higher income have shorter waiting times for diagnosis visits in publicly-funded systems, and that patients with lower level of education wait longer relative to those with higher educational attainments. Using survey data from Italy, Landi, Ivaldi and Testi (2018[17]) found that low education and income are associated with a higher risk of experiencing long waiting times for diagnostic and specialist visits.

3.3. Waiting times may worsen health outcomes

Beyond concerns about inequalities, another concern with rationing through waiting times is that the wait may worsen health outcomes for patients before and after the intervention. The evidence shows that this depends on the duration of the wait, the health problem (whether or not physical or mental health is likely to deteriorate quickly), and the ability of clinicians to prioritise.

A review of the literature for coronary bypass suggests that long waits may worsen symptoms and clinical outcomes following the operation (Sobolev and Fradet, 2008[18]). Waiting may also increase the probability of pre-operative death (while waiting) and unplanned emergency admission (Sobolev and Fradet, 2008[18]; Sobolev et al., 2012[19]). However, Moscelli, Siciliani and Tonei (2016[20]) did not find any evidence in England that waiting times for elective coronary bypass was associated with higher in-hospital mortality and only a weak association between waiting times and emergency readmission following a surgery.

Nikolova, Harrison and Sutton (2016[21]) found that long waits for patients in England on the waiting lists for common elective procedures reduce their health-related quality of life for hip and knee replacement while they are waiting, but not for other interventions such as varicose veins and inguinal hernia.

A review of the literature for mental health services found some evidence showing that shorter waiting times can have a positive effect on outcomes. Early access to services for some conditions, such as psychosis, has been shown to have a strong therapeutic benefit (Bird et al., 2010[22]; Reichert and Jacobs, 2018[23]). Similar impacts have been observed for children and adolescents seeking mental health services, where longer wait times can contribute to a higher rate of 'no shows', greater likelihood of disengaging from services during the therapeutic process, and possible worsening of the condition (Schraeder and Reid, 2015[24]; Westin, Barksdale and Stephan, 2014[25]; Kowalewski, McLennan and McGrath, 2011[26]).

Reducing psychiatric waiting times could also lead to efficiency gains and cost savings. A study in Los Angeles in a community mental health centre serving 30 000 people found that more rapid access to psychiatric services had positive impacts including 'no shows' to appointments falling by more than half – estimated to have led to cost savings of USD 44 000 in psychiatrist time – and reduced crisis hospitalisations (Williams, Latta and Conversano, 2008[27]). Where waiting for treatment is associated with deterioration in the person's condition, there may be other economic costs, for example if the patient has poorer outcomes from treatment after having waited an extended period (Reichert and Jacobs, 2018[23]), or if their worsened condition prevents them from working (OECD, 2012[28]; Royal College of Psychiatrists, 2018[29]).

People seeking mental health support have also reported distress at long waiting lists for services, and being unable to access care in a timely way (Government Inquiry into Mental Health and Addiction, 2018[30]; Biringer et al., 2015[31]).

4 Policies to address waiting times can target the supply side, the demand side, or both

Policies to reduce waiting times can increase supply, reduce or better manage demand, or both (Box 4.1). The most common policy remains the introduction of a maximum waiting time, which can be used to mobilise efforts to bring together the supply and demand in a variety of ways. It can be used by governments to establish some overall objective or target for various health services at the system level. It can also be used as a target at the provider level or to give patients a guarantee that treatment will be given within a certain time limit. When waiting times are specified as a target, regulators and funders may use it as an accountability measure for providers, with possible consequences when the target is not met. When maximum waiting times are specified as a guarantee, they can be enforced through the law or provide patients with the right to change provider. If not specified as a target, a guarantee or linked to specific actions, maximum waiting times act more as an ambition than a policy lever.

Box 4.1. Several demand-side and supply-side factors affect waiting times

Waiting times are a dynamic phenomenon. They increase over time if demand exceeds the supply, and reduce if supply exceeds demand. Both demand and supply are likely to grow over time. Demand increases over time because of population ageing, which increases needs, or through technological development, which increases the range of conditions that are treatable. Supply may also increase over time due to technological development, which for example allows patients to be treated as day cases in hospitals, possibly allowing a larger number of patients to be treated over a given week or month. This dynamic element implies that periods of increasing supply can be associated with increasing waiting times if demand grows at a faster rate.

The demand for treatments in public systems is also determined by other factors beyond ageing and technology, such as patient preferences for surgery, patient cost-sharing (e.g. co-payments, coinsurance rates), the extent to which the population holds (duplicative) private health insurance and the price and accessibility of private care (Figure 4.1).

The supply of treatments is determined by the overall capacity which depends on the health workforce and its composition, and infrastructure and equipment (e.g. number of primary care facilities, clinics and hospitals, and diagnostic and surgical equipment). However, it is not only the availability of labour and capital, but also the productivity with which the capacity is used that determines the supply. Productivity will depend on contractual arrangements with health workers (hours, number of sessions) and payment systems (e.g. for doctors and nurses) and at the organisation level (hospital and primary care facilities). Incentives to increase supply are stronger when health workers are paid by fee for service as opposed to salaried or capitation, and provider payments are based on activities, although this might also generate some supply-induced demand.

Figure 4.1. Conceptual framework to analyse waiting lists and waiting times for elective care

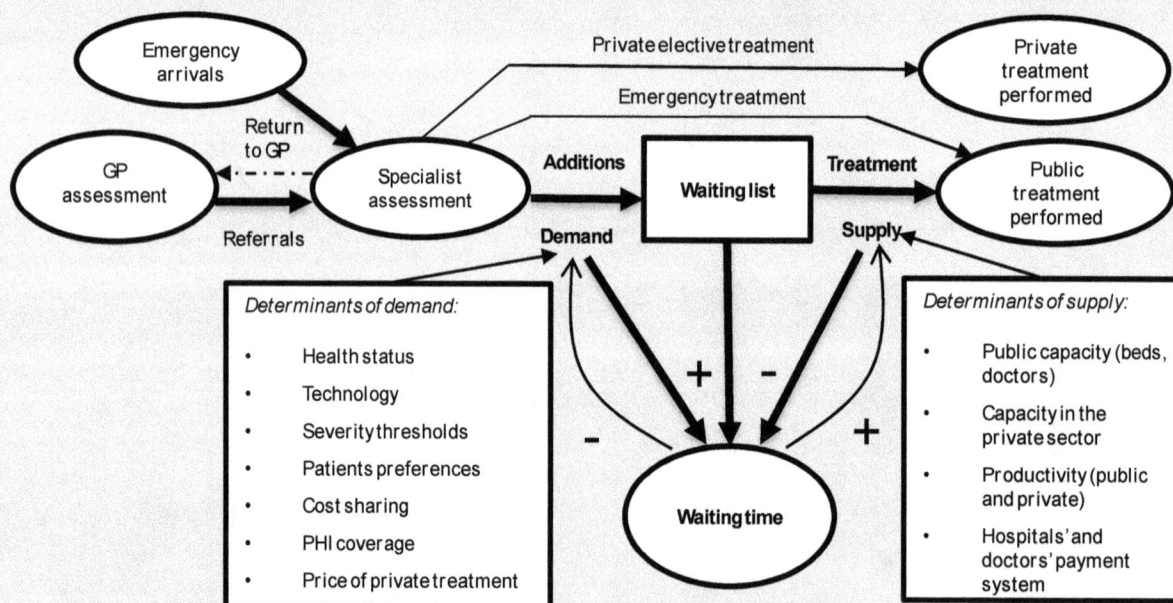

Source: Adapted from Hurst and Siciliani (2003[32]), "Tackling Excessive Waiting Times for Elective Surgery: A Comparison of Policies in Twelve OECD Countries", *OECD Health Working Papers*, No. 6, https://doi.org/10.1787/108471127058.

As shown in Figure 4.1, a number of supply-side policies can be used to reduce waiting times, with the most common ones being to increase resources (human and/or technical) and productivity. Other policies act on the demand side, mostly aiming at prioritising patients based on need to avoid adding them to the waiting list when there is little or no expected benefits, reducing inappropriate referrals, tests and procedures, or redistributing waiting times across patients with different severity (so that patients with more severe conditions wait less).

The next sections review maximum waiting times that OECD countries have set and some of the main policy actions on the supply and the demand side to achieve these goals in four clinical areas:

1. Specialist consultations and elective treatments;
2. Consultations with GPs and other primary care providers;
3. Cancer care (diagnosis and treatment); and
4. Mental health services (diagnosis and treatment).

4.1. Policies to reduce waiting times for specialist consultations and elective treatments

The most common policy used across OECD countries to reduce waiting times for specialist consultations and elective treatments is to establish a maximum waiting time. As illustrated in Table 4.1, maximum waiting times vary across countries. Some countries specify maximum waiting times only for specific treatments, others for all treatments. The segment of the patient pathway over which the maximum applies also differs. Most countries have a maximum wait specified for an elective treatment following a specialist assessment, yet others specify it from the GP referral to treatment. Others also have a maximum waiting time for specialist consultations and diagnostic tests. The same maximum waiting time can apply to all the patients within the same type of service, or different maximum can be applied to different sub-groups, usually in relation to clinical categorisation and severity of conditions.

Maximum waiting times for the same service or treatment can differ extensively across countries, which may in part reflect different constraints on funding and resources. For example, the maximum waiting time for a cataract surgery ranges from one month in Denmark to 1.5 years in Estonia. Regarding consultations with specialists, it ranges from 3 weeks in Finland up to a target that 80% of patients should get a first outpatient appointment with a specialist within 52 weeks in Ireland.

Table 4.1. Maximum waiting times for specialist consultations and elective treatments

Country	Maximum waiting times
Australia	Clinical urgency categorisation: • Category 1: 30 days (patient's health has the potential to deteriorate quickly) • Category 2: 90 days (patient's health not likely to deteriorate quickly) • Category 3: 365 days (patient's health unlikely to deteriorate quickly)
Canada	• Hip and knee replacement: 26 weeks • Cataract surgery: 16 weeks • Cancer care - Radiation therapy: 4 weeks • Cardiac care - Bypass surgery: range from 2 to 26 weeks depending on urgency
Czech Republic	• Hip and knee replacement: 52 weeks • Cataract surgery: 30 weeks • Angiography non-coronary arteries and vascular intervention: 8 weeks
Denmark	• Extended free hospital choice means you have the right to receive examination or treatment in a private hospital if you have to wait more than 30 days

Country	Maximum waiting times
Estonia	• Outpatient consultation/visit: 6 weeks • Inpatient specialist care and day care: 8 months • Cataract surgery, hip and knee replacement and other elective surgery: 1.5 year
Finland	• Specialist assessment: 3 weeks • Maximum waiting time (guarantee): 3 months (may be extended 6 months)
Hungary	• Minor surgery: 60 days • Major surgery: 180 days
Iceland	• Specialist visit: 30 days • For 80% of patients, diagnosis to treatment: 90 days
Ireland	• 90% of children wait less than 15 months for an elective inpatient or day case procedure • 90% of adults wait less than 15 months for an elective inpatient procedure • 95% of adults wait less than 15 months for an elective day case procedure • 80% of patients waiting for a first outpatient appointment will be seen within 52 weeks
Latvia	• Specialists consultations for persons with a predictable disability: 15 working days • Surgical manipulations: 5 months
Lithuania	• Specialist consultation/visit: 30 calendar days • Inpatient, day-case, day-surgery services: 60 calendar days
Netherlands	• Specialist visit and diagnostic: 4 weeks • Outpatient care: 4 weeks • Inpatient treatment: 7 weeks
New Zealand	• Receipt of referral to First Specialist Assessment: 4 months • Patient acceptance to treatment: 120 days
Norway	• All patients with a right to specialised treatment are given an individually assessed deadline • In addition, there is an overall goal of reducing average waiting times below 50 days by 2021
Portugal	• Visit (normal priority level): 120 days • Treatment (normal priority level): 180 days
Spain (different regions)	Pais Vasco and Baleares: • Specialist visits : 30 days • Elective treatment: 180 days Cantabria: • Specialist visit: 60 days Madrid: • Specialist visit: 60 days • Elective treatment: 180 days Murcia: • Specialist visit: 50 days Navarra: • Specialist visit: Ordinarily less than 30 business days, preferred less than 10 business days • Elective treatment (depends on the procedure): 30 days (cancer surgery), 60 days (cardiac surgery), 120 days and 180 days (if the wait does not mean worsening of health)
United Kingdom	• At least 92% patients referred to see a consultant-led team start their treatment within 18 weeks

Note: There can also be other targets for disease-specific pathways (i.e. cancer or cardiac care pathways).
Source: OECD Waiting Times questionnaire 2019.

While all these countries start by setting maximum waiting time targets for specialist consultations and/or elective treatments, the way these maximums are used differs significantly across countries. The description of the policies across the OECD countries fall in five categories:

1. Maximum waiting times targets for providers (e.g. Finland, England)

2. Maximum waiting times guarantees allowing greater patient choice of providers (e.g. Denmark and Portugal)

3. Increased supply to achieve progress towards maximum waiting time objectives (e.g. the Netherlands, Ireland, Canada, Costa Rica)

4. Improving demand management by prioritising patients on the list (e.g. New Zealand, Norway)

5. Improved coordination between primary and secondary care to reduce unnecessary referrals to specialists and waiting times for specialist assessment when needed (e.g. New Zealand, Canada, Italy).

It is important to recognise that these groups are not mutually exclusive ant that each country may have introduced elements of different policies at the same time or may have changed their policy mix over time.

4.1.1. Maximum waiting times have been used as a target for providers in Finland and the United Kingdom and can be successful in reducing waiting times through supply and demand side responses

Both Finland and England have used maximum waiting times as targets for providers or in the case of Finland for municipalities, with sanctions for providers not making progress towards the targets in some cases and strong regulatory oversight. The introduction of these policies has been successful in reducing waiting times significantly starting from very high levels in both countries.

In **Finland**, some maximum waiting times for specialist consultation and elective treatment were specified as targets in 2005 as part the broader Health Care Guarantee. It was then included into legislation through the Finnish Health Care Act in 2010. The Act stated that patients should have a specialist consultation within 3 weeks following a referral from a GP or other primary care providers; for elective surgery, any evaluation should occur within three weeks, and diagnostic tests within 3 months; and if surgery is needed, this should normally occur within 3 months from the assessment but can be extended to 6 months for non-urgent interventions. A regulatory agency (the National Supervisory Agency Valvira) played a key role in supervising the implementation of these waiting times guarantees and had the authority to penalise municipalities that failed to meet them. It provided targets to municipalities for progressive reductions in the number of patients waiting over 6 months, and by early 2012 had issued 30 orders for improvement, including 8 with a threat of fines (Siciliani, Borowitz and Moran, 2013[1]).The introduction of the guarantee led to a significant decline in waiting times for elective surgery starting in 2005, which has been sustained since then (Figure 4.2).[4]

Figure 4.2. Following the introduction of maximum waiting times in 2005, waiting times for elective surgery have reduced in Finland

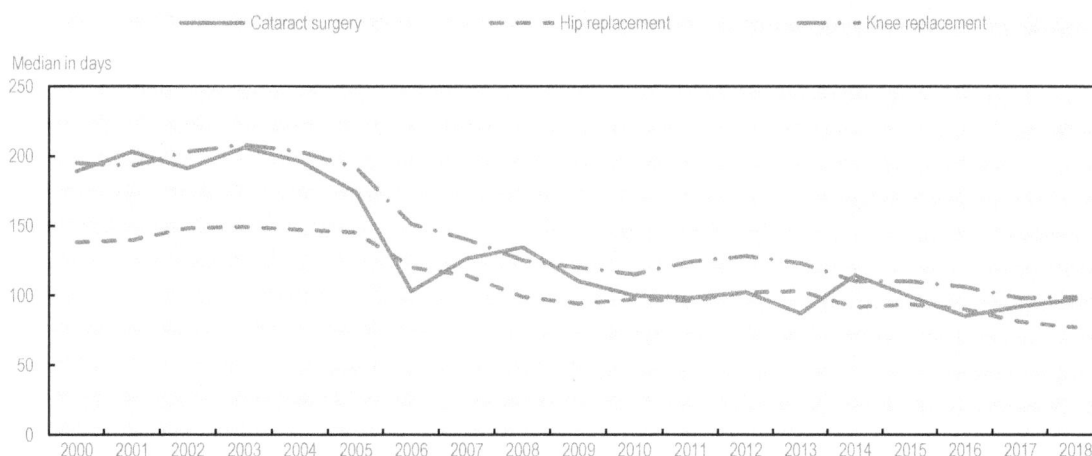

Source: OECD Health Statistics.

The policy emphasis in Finland has been on setting and achieving the maximum waiting times targets, with providers and municipalities responsible to implement policies and actions (either on the supply- or the demand side) to achieve these targets.

Figure 4.3 shows that the supply of elective operations continued to increase after 2005. This suggests that the reductions in waiting times were achieved by a mix of supply-side measures and better management of the demand. Although Finland has managed to maintain the reduction in waiting times after 2005, waiting times are still relatively high compared to other countries like Denmark and there is scope for further reductions (Figure 2.3).

Figure 4.3. Growing volumes of elective surgery have contributed to the reduction in waiting times in Finland since 2005

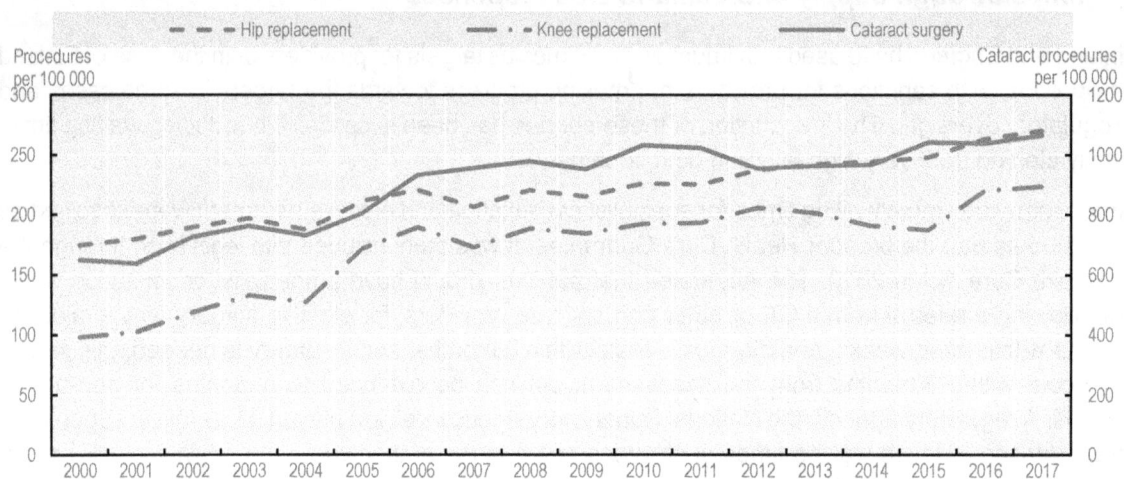

Source: OECD Health Statistics.

In **England**, maximum waiting time guarantees were set respectively at 12 months in 2002-03 and 9 months in 2003-04, and then progressively reduced to 18 weeks by 2006. Targets with penalties were introduced in 2000-05, with strong political oversight from the Prime Ministerial Delivery Unit and the Health Care Commission. These contributed to dramatic reductions in waiting times for several elective surgeries between 2000 and 2008. The median waiting times was cut down by more than half for hip and knee replacement as well as for cataract surgery (Figure 4.4).

Figure 4.4. Waiting times for elective surgery have reduced sharply in the United Kingdom in the previous decade and have been generally stable since 2008

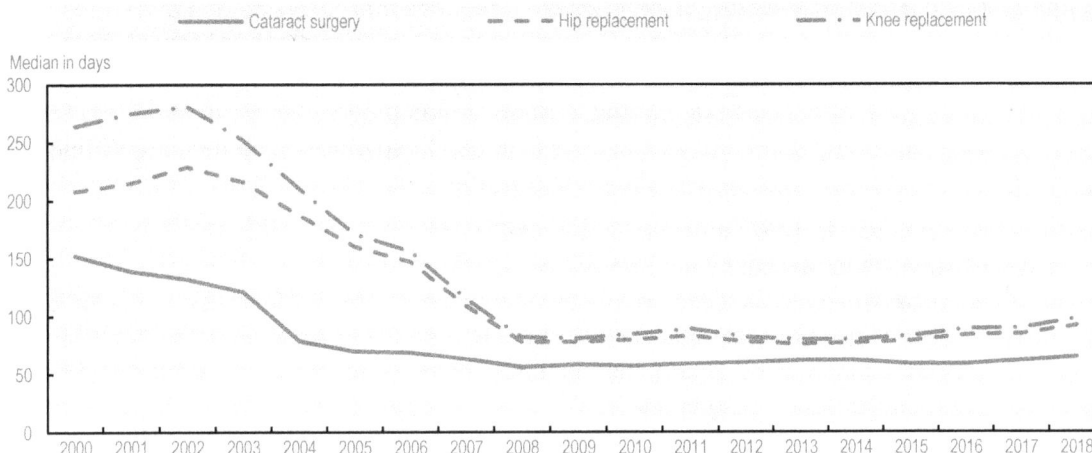

Note: The data relate to Great Britain (England, Scotland and Wales).
Source: OECD Health Statistics.

As has been the case in Finland, the reduction in waiting times for both knee and hip replacement between 2000 and 2008, and to some extent also cataract surgery, is partly linked to an increase in surgical activity rates (Figure 4.5), though the very sharp reductions in waiting times during that period (relative to the following period from 2009-18) suggest that better management of demand also played a role.

Figure 4.5. Growing surgical activity rates have contributed to the reduction in waiting times in the United Kingdom in the previous decade

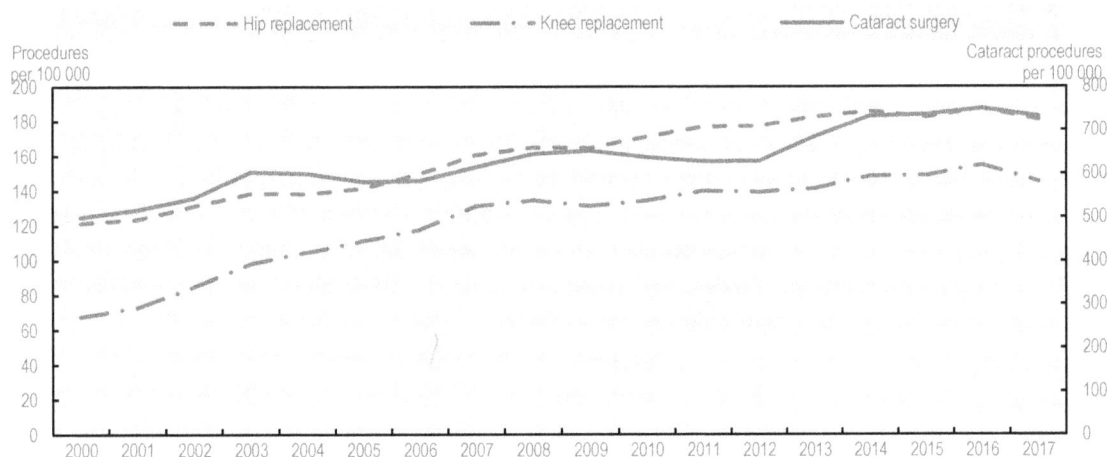

Source: OECD Health Statistics.

In 2010, waiting times guarantees were codified into the NHS Constitution, where patient entitlement to the 18 weeks maximum referred to the waiting time between GP referral to treatment (RTT). The RTT standard is set out in secondary legislation (The National Health Service Commissioning Board and Clinical Commissioning Groups (CCG) Regulations 2012). It requires that NHS England and CCGs make arrangements to ensure that at least 92% patients referred to see a consultant-led team should start their treatment within 18 weeks. In 2013, about 94% of patients on the list (known as "incomplete pathway") were waiting less than 18 weeks, but this proportion has progressively decreased to 86% in 2018, which has coincided with a period of slower growth in health spending. The median waiting time has increased from 5.6 weeks in April 2013 to 7.2 in April 2019.

The Long-Term Plan commits to help reduce waiting times against this standard. The Plan includes a reform of outpatient services to: a) reduce the number of appointments with specialists that may not be needed; and b) increase variety of access to appointments (e.g. through increased use of digital services). There are also plans to allocate sufficient funds over the next years to increase the volume of planned surgery and reduce long waits. Again, these interventions reflect a mix of demand and supply measures to achieve reductions in waiting times.

4.1.2. Maximum waiting times have been linked to greater patient choice of provider with some degree of success in Denmark and Portugal

Two countries, Denmark and Portugal, have linked maximum waiting times with patient choice policies and some involvement of the private sector when waiting times reach certain levels. These policies have contributed to reductions in waiting times in Denmark that have been sustained over time, while reductions in waiting times were achieved initially in Portugal but have proven more difficult to sustain in recent years. The reductions in waiting times in Denmark are smaller relative to those obtained in Finland and England, which is also due to the much lower initial levels.

Since 2002, patients in **Denmark** are guaranteed a maximum waiting time from a GP or specialist referral to treatment, initially set at two months but then reduced to one month in 2007. If the region cannot ensure that treatment will be initiated within one month, patients have the right to some 'extended free choice of hospital'. This means that patients may choose to go to a private hospital in Denmark or to a public or private hospital abroad. If the treatment is provided outside of the region's own hospitals, the expenses are covered by the originating region through a DRG tariff, thereby providing incentives for regions to keep patients within the county. Waiting time declined after 2002, with the proportion of patients using private sector providers under free choice increasing from 2% to about 5% between 2006 and 2010 (Siciliani, Borowitz and Moran, 2013[1]). Figure 4.6 shows that the reduction in waiting times for selected surgical procedures has been achieved between 2005 and 2018, but with some fluctuations from year-to-year. As shown in Figure 2.3, waiting times are generally low relative to other countries (about 2 to 6 weeks depending on the procedure), despite a definition of waiting time that is broader and includes the time from a GP or specialist referral to treatment.

Figure 4.6. Waiting times for elective surgery have reduced in Denmark since 2005

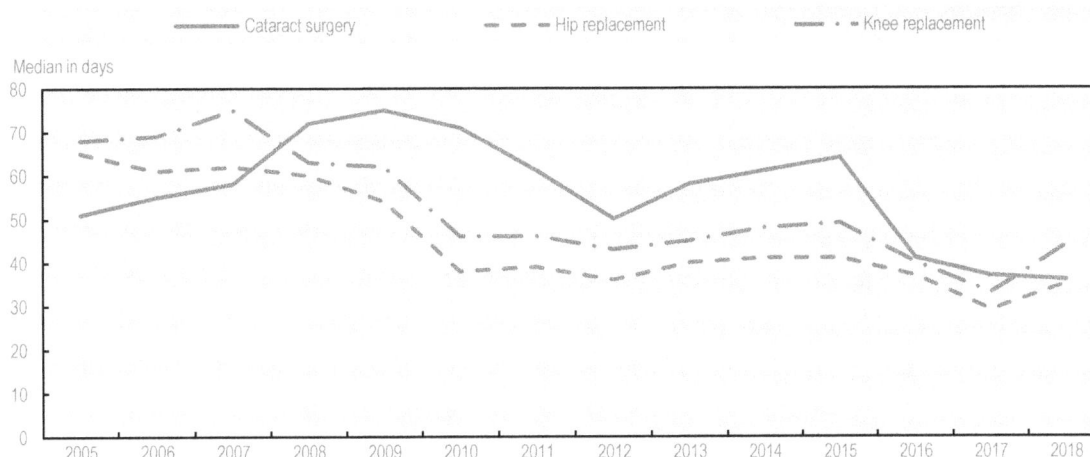

Note: Waiting times for some elective surgery like cataract operations increased in 2008 and 2009 because a hospital dispute in May 2008 led to the postponement of all non-urgent operations, which were rescheduled after the summer 2008. By the end of the dispute, a substantial backlog had built up, which took some time for hospitals to clear.
Source: OECD Health Statistics.

The extended free patient choice policy still holds and also applies to hospital referrals. The regions are required to ensure that any patient referred to a hospital is assessed within one month from the date of referral. If, for medical reasons, it is not possible to determine the condition of the patient within one month, the patient must receive a detailed plan to ensure further investigation of his/her health problem (including, for example, further examinations at another hospital). If because of limited capacity, the region is not able to provide such an assessment within 30 days, the extended free choice of hospital applies (i.e. the patient may go to a private hospital or a hospital abroad to be diagnosed).

After several policies that involved additional funding with limited effects, **Portugal** introduced in 2004 a policy combining a new mandatory integrated information system (known as the SIGIC) with waiting time guarantees. This policy also involved a voucher system such that when the patient on the list reaches 75% of the maximum time, a voucher is issued that allows the patient to seek treatment at any provider, including in the private sector. Between 2005 and 2010, the national waiting list for surgery declined by 39% (Siciliani, Borowitz and Moran, 2013[1]), and the median waiting times for selected elective surgeries also declined (Figure 4.7).

However, some of these earlier reductions have not been sustained in recent years, and waiting times have increased again since 2011. The average waiting time for surgical treatments was 2.9 months in 2015 and slowly increasing to 3.3 months in 2018. This is despite a 6% growth in surgery over this period (from about 560 000 to 595 000), but this fell short of the 7% increase in the number of people that were added to the waiting list (which rose from about 660 000 to 705 000) (OECD waiting time policy questionnaire, 2019).

Figure 4.7. Waiting times for elective surgery have increased in Portugal since 2011, following a reduction in the previous decade

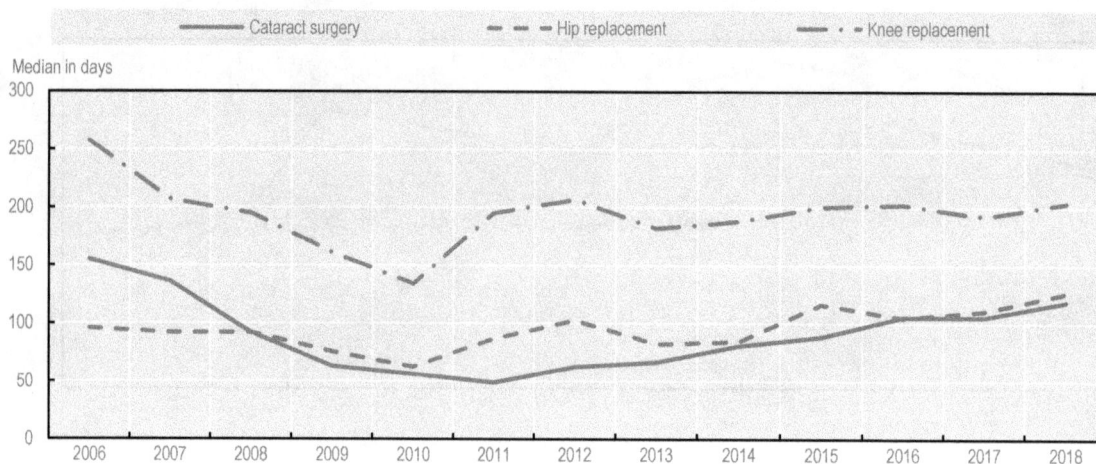

Source: OECD Health Statistics.

SIGIC is being replaced with a new information system, SIGA (Access to Healthcare Integrated System), which is more patient-centred. It provides a horizontal and integrated approach to monitor waiting times along the patient pathway in five phases: Phase 1 – Referral from hospital to primary care; Phase 2 – Referral from primary care to hospital; Phase 3 – Referral intra and inter hospitals; Phase 4 – Referral from NHS contact centre to hospitals and primary care; and Phase 5 – Referral to and from the National Network of Long-Term Care. The current maximum waiting times for elective treatment is 180 days (for normal priority level), 120 days for specialist visits and 90 days for diagnostic tests such an MRI or a CT scan. Other initiatives under the "Access to healthcare improvement plan" include improving the prioritisation of the waiting list by setting waiting times based on clinical priority, benchmarking, and improved coordination protocols between hospitals and primary care units.

Since 2016, there is "Free Circulation of Patients" for specialist visits with patients being offered the possibility to choose another hospital in the NHS to the one they are regularly referred to. In consultation with the GP, patients can choose the hospital taking into account the waiting times published in the NHS portal (http://tempos.min-saude.pt/#/instituicoes), which provides waiting times also for surgery.

4.1.3. Many countries focus on increasing supply as the main policy lever to reduce waiting times, but these can be expensive or not successful in achieving lasting reductions

Several countries (e.g. the Netherlands, Ireland, Australia, Canada, Hungary, Estonia, Poland and Slovenia) have tried to reduce waiting times mainly by increasing the supply of services and procedures with different degrees of success, and many other countries are planning to introduce such measures. Supply can be increased through dedicated funding, by inducing doctors and other members of health care teams to do additional sessions and longer hours, and by recruiting additional staff. This policy is expensive and will lead to reductions in waiting only if the increase in supply outweighs the increase in demand, and if the health system does not respond to higher volumes by a commensurate increase in referrals and procedures that inflates demand (a form of supply-induced demand). Supply can also be increased through greater efficiency of the operating theatre and work organisation.

In the **Netherlands**, the national associations of hospitals and insurers agreed in 2000 on a socially acceptable waiting time (known as "Treek norms") of six weeks (80% within four weeks) for day treatment and seven weeks (80% within five weeks) for in-patient treatment, and four weeks (80% within three weeks) for hospital specialist diagnosis and medical assessment. This was also motivated by a court decision stating that patients had an enforceable right to timely health care.

Several initiatives to increase the supply of services were introduced at the same time. In 2001, hospital reimbursement changed from fixed budget to activity-based payments, and restrictions on the number of medical specialists in hospitals were abolished. Waiting times decreased substantially to about 5 weeks on average for cataract surgery in 2010 and 7 weeks for hip and knee replacement (Figure 4.8), down from over 12 weeks for these three interventions in 2000 (Siciliani, Borowitz and Moran, 2013[1]). This was linked at least partly to an increase in surgical activities during that period (Figure 4.9). Waiting times remained low until 2013-14 but have since then started to increase again, possibly due to the re-introduction of budget caps that has limited the supply in the face of growing demand.

Figure 4.8. Waiting times for elective surgery have started to go up in the Netherlands since 2015

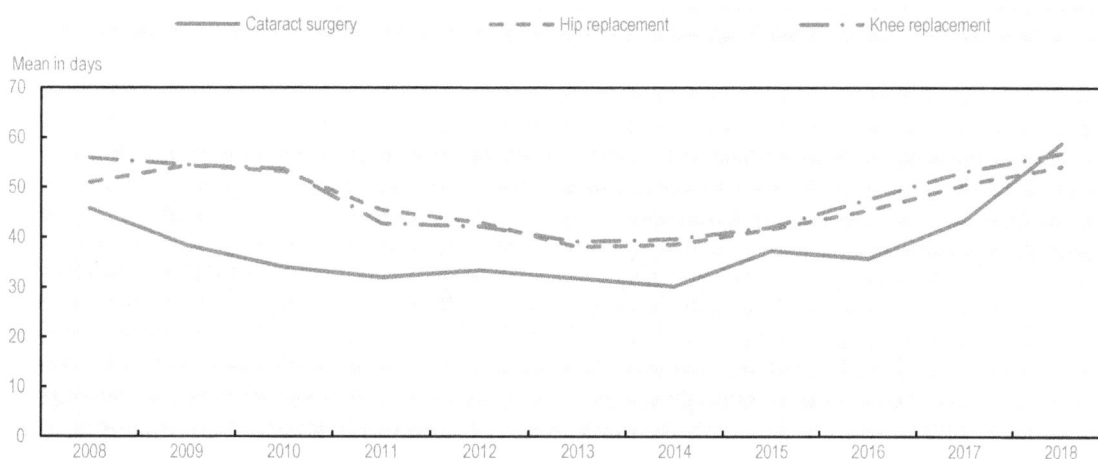

Note: The data start in 2008 because there is a break in the series in that year.
Source: OECD Health Statistics.

Figure 4.9. Growing volumes of elective surgery contributed to the reduction in waiting times in the Netherlands until recently

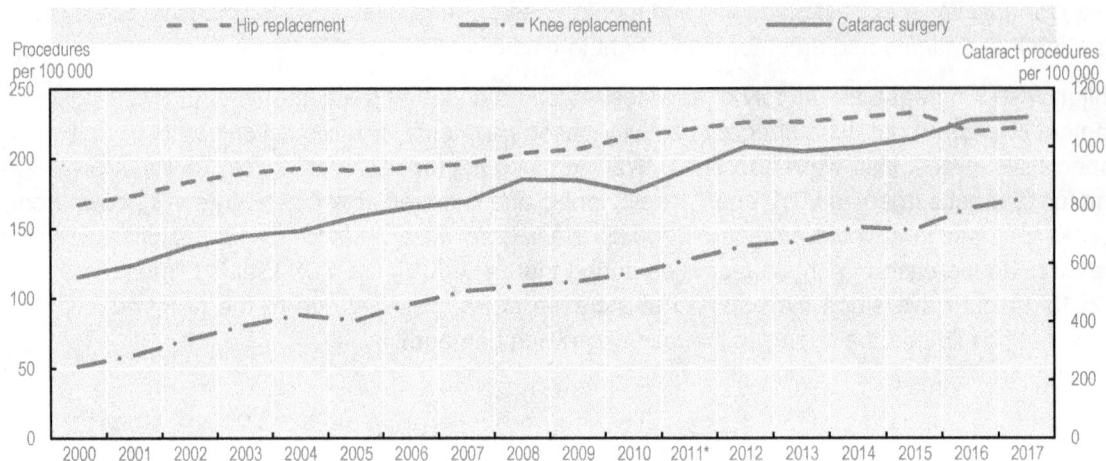

Note: There is a data gap for all procedures in 2011, which has been estimated as the average of surgical activity rates in 2010 and 2012.
Source: OECD Health Statistics 2019.

Ireland has also introduced many maximum waiting times targets and supply-side measures to try to reduce long waiting times for different health services, including specialist consultations and elective surgery, with uneven success. The National Service Plan increased the funding available to the Health Service Executive (HSE) by an average of 5% per year in 2018 and 2019 to respond to growing demands for health care, including specialist care and elective care, following substantial increases between 2012 and 2017. The increased funding and activities has contributed to a reduction in waiting times in 2018, with the number and share of patients waiting over 3 months falling significantly in 2018 (Figure 4.10). This has also been the case for the number of patients waiting over 9 months, which has come down from 28 100 in July 2017 to 14 900 at the end of 2018. By the end of 2018, 84% (93%) of adults waited less than 15 months for an elective inpatient (day case) procedure, which falls short of the targets of 90% (and 95%); and 90% (84%) of children waited less than 15 months for an elective inpatient (day case) procedure, falling short of the 90% target for day cases; 70% of patients were waiting less than 52 weeks for first outpatient appointment. While waiting times for elective surgery has started to come down in 2018, they remain higher than in 2012, and generally waiting times in Ireland remain high relatively to many other OECD countries (Figure 2.3).

Figure 4.10. Following increases in previous years, waiting times for elective surgery in Ireland have started to come down in 2018

% of patients on the waiting list for over 3 months

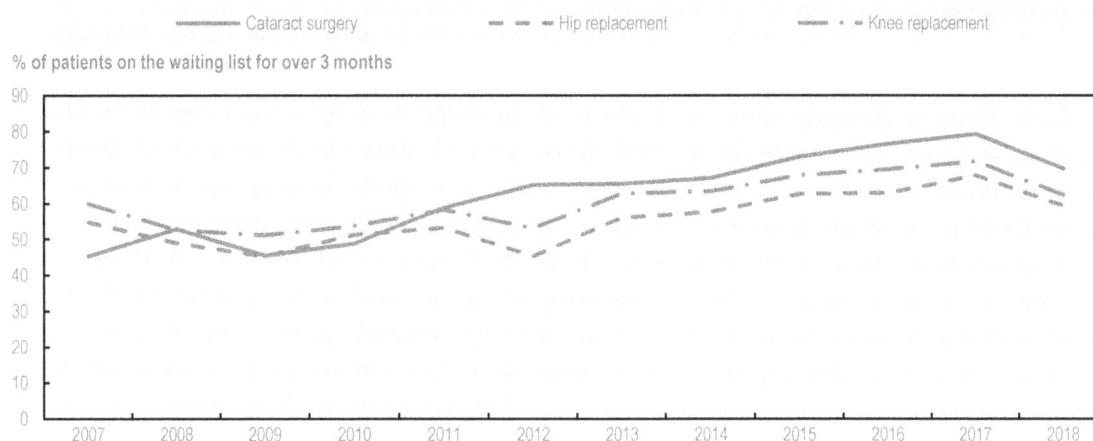

Source: National Treatment Purchase Fund (the data refer to the situation in mid-year, end of June).

The objective in 2019 is to further reduce the number of patients waiting longer than 3 (9) months from 40 200 (14 900) at the end of 2018 to 31 000 (10 000) at the end of 2019. The Department of Health oversees the performance of the HSE and the National Treatment Purchase Fund (NTPF) against agreed targets. This includes weekly analysis of waiting list figures provided by the NTPF and regular review meetings with the HSE and the NTPF. The Department of Health has also convened a Working Group to examine current and projected demand and capacity to deliver services, with a view to improve access to elective care in the short, medium, and long term in different specialty areas (e.g. orthopaedics, dermatology, ophthalmology, urology and gynaecology).

In **Australia**, the 2011-15 National Partnership Agreement on Improving Public Hospital Services between the Australian Government and all states and territories agreed on some National Elective Surgery Targets as well as a National Emergency Access Target. States and territories received additional government funding to improve facilities and undertake process redesign, and reward payments if they met or partially met the agreed-upon targets each year. The former Council of Australian Governments (COAG) reported publicly on the progress of states and territories towards achieving these targets. In its last report from 2014, it found that no state or territory met all their 2013 elective surgery targets, though some were met.

The dedicated investments in elective surgery during the term of the 2011-15 Agreement were only sufficient to meet the growing demand, without any significant impact in reducing waiting times. Between 2015 and 2018, waiting times for cataract surgery have declined slightly, but they have increased slightly for knee replacement and hip replacement (Figure 4.11). Although Australia does not currently have a national policy to reduce waiting times for elective surgery, the government still regularly evaluates waiting times in public hospitals based on nationally agreed performance indicators on waiting times. The Australian Institute of Health and Welfare compiles the data provided by the states and territories to produce the Australian hospital statistics series of annual reports.

Figure 4.11. Waiting times for cataract surgery have come down slightly in Australia since 2015, but they have gone up for knee replacement

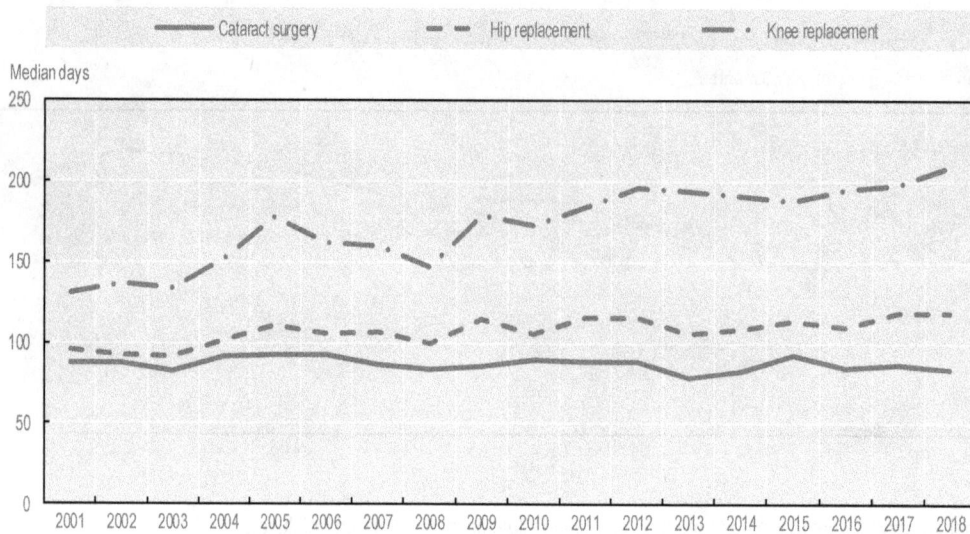

Source: OECD Health Statistics.

In **Canada**, federal, provincial and territorial governments committed in 2004 on a ten-year plan to reduce waiting times for some elective surgery, including cataract and hip and knee replacement and to improve the reporting of waiting times data. Between 2008 and 2014, the median waiting times for these three elective surgical procedures remained relatively stable, but they have increased since 2014 (Figure 4.12). The demand for these procedures has increased more rapidly than the number of surgeries due to population ageing as well as increases in the prevalence of conditions such as osteoarthritis and obesity (CIHI, 2019[33]). The province of British Columbia in Canada announced in 2018 that it would be completing approximately 9 400 more surgeries in the public health care system by March 2019, with a focus on improving surgical pathways, coordination of care and information to patients.

Figure 4.12. Waiting times for elective surgery have increased in Canada since 2014

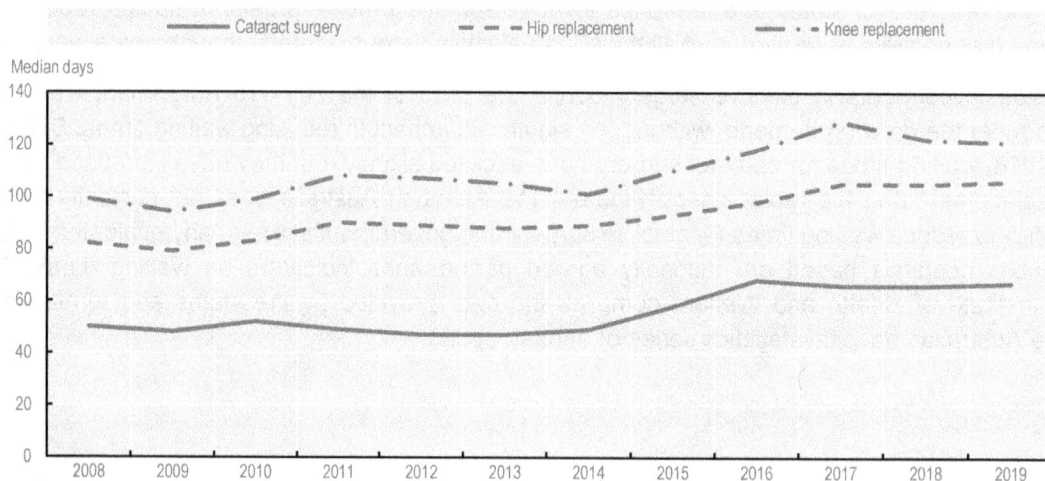

Source: OECD Health Statistics.

Hungary has achieved progress in reducing waiting times for elective surgery over the past five years through the implementation of its 2014-2020 strategy for the health sector, which includes supply-side measures along with better management of demand (Figure 4.13). As a result, waiting times for elective surgery in Hungary is much lower than in all other Central and Eastern European countries that report these data (Figure 2.3).

One of the main objectives of the 2014-2020 strategy is to reduce waiting times to less than 60 days for minor surgery (like cataract surgery) and less than 180 days for major surgery (like hip and knee replacement) for all patients across the country. This involves efforts to reduce regional inequalities in timely access of elective care. To achieve this goal, the government has adopted new laws and regulations regarding the management of waiting lists, that are supported by the development of an online waiting list system at the national level to monitor the situation in real-time. It also provided additional payments to reduce waiting times in selected clinical areas and hospitals, and encouraged a reallocation of patients from providers with longer waiting times to those with shorter waiting times.

Figure 4.13. Waiting times for elective surgery have decreased in Hungary since 2015

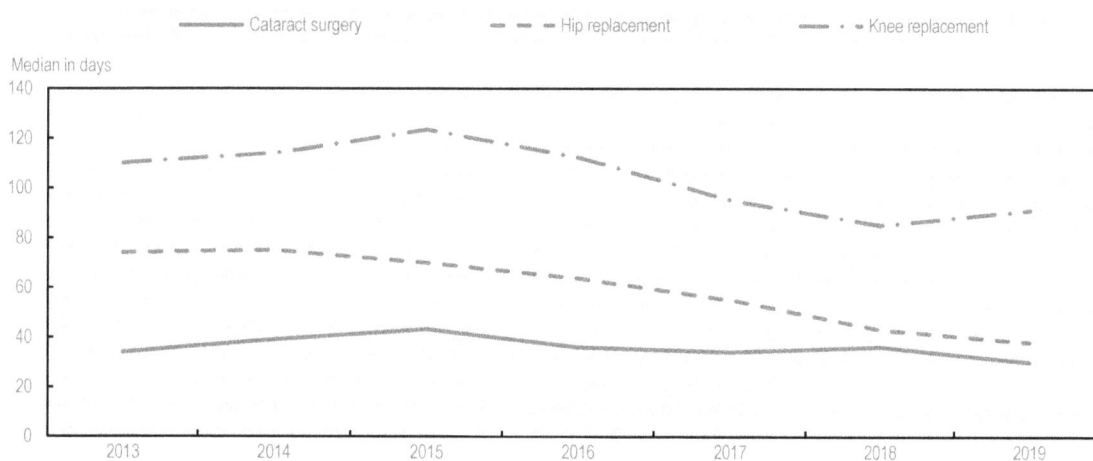

Source: OECD Health Statistics.

Estonia is a country where waiting times for elective strategy have traditionally been long. Between 2007 and 2014, a marked reduction in waiting times for cataract surgery and joint replacement was achieved, due at least partly to additional funding provided in some years to increase surgical activity rates. The waiting time guarantee for hip and knee replacement was also shortened from 2.5 years to 1.5 years at the beginning of 2013. However, since 2014, waiting times for these elective surgery have started to go up again, returning to their level of 2007 in the case of hip replacement or to even higher level in the case of knee replacement (Figure 4.14). In 2018, the Health Insurance Fund provided an additional EUR 34 million to improve the availability of specialist services and finance about 140 000 additional treatments. The goal was to reduce waiting times for cataract surgery and joint replacement. The number of these operations increased substantially over the previous years (Figure 4.15). This was accompanied by a reduction in waiting times for cataract surgery and hip replacement, but not for knee replacement.

Figure 4.14. Waiting times for elective surgery decreased sharply in Estonia until 2015, but have increased since then

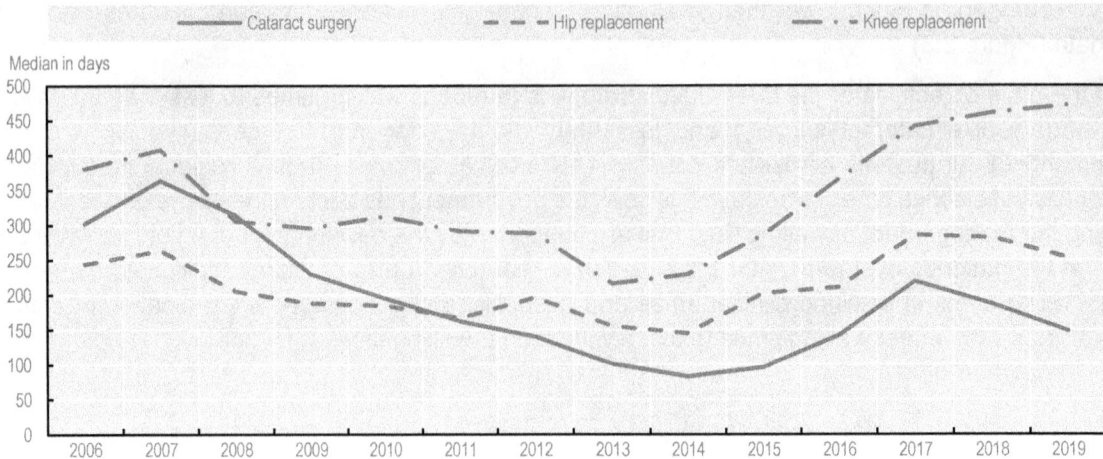

Source: OECD Health Statistics.

Figure 4.15. The volume of cataract surgery and joint replacement increased greatly in Estonia in 2018 to reduce waiting times

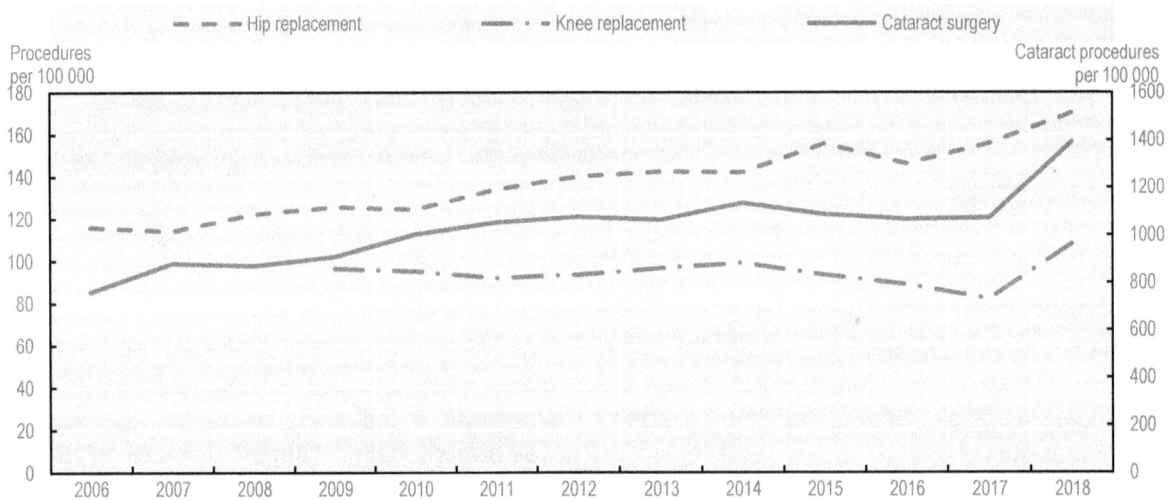

Source: OECD Health Statistics.

Poland has also taken steps to increase the supply of elective care to reduce waiting times. Waiting times for cataract surgery and joint replacement started to fall in 2018 (Figure 4.16) as the number of these surgical procedures increased substantially (Figure 4.17). Until 2018, if the demand for services exceeded what had been budgeted for, elective services were rationed through waiting lists with the services postponed to the next year. Since 2018, additional funding is provided for additional treatments, targeting a reduction in waiting times for cataract surgery, and hip and knee replacement. Information on waiting times for different treatments in public hospitals are now also more easily accessible to patients through a dedicated website. A growing number of Polish people also purchase a private health insurance to get quicker access to services in private hospitals.

Figure 4.16. Waiting times for elective surgery decreased sharply in Poland in 2018

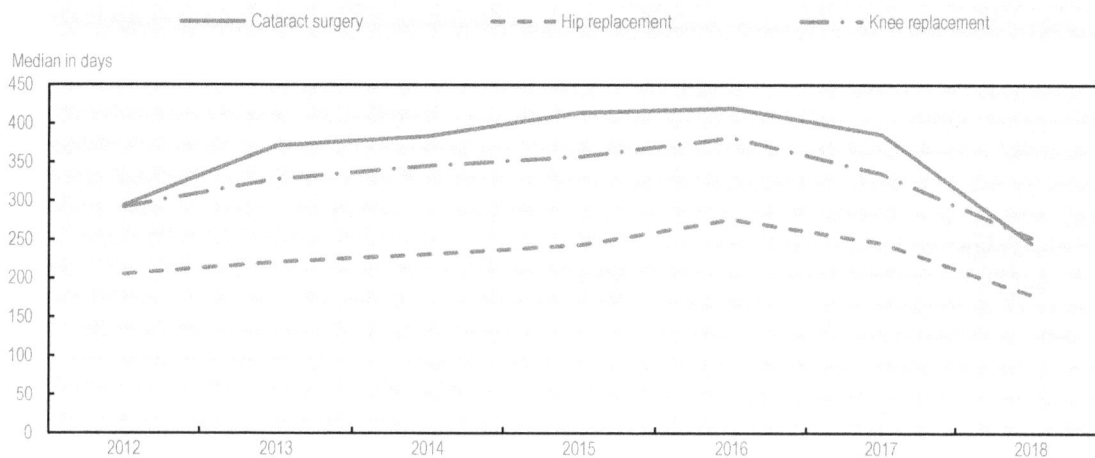

Note: These data only relate to waiting times in public hospitals.
Source: OECD Health Statistics.

Figure 4.17. The volume of cataract surgery and joint replacement has increased substantially in Poland in recent years

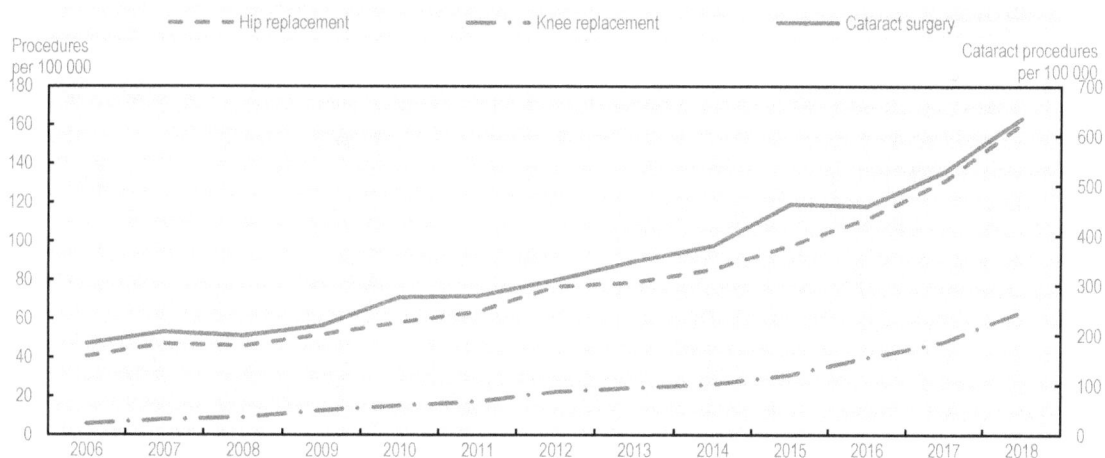

Source: OECD Health Statistics.

In **Slovenia**, additional financial resources in 2016-18 were earmarked to increase services with excessive waiting times. Moreover, some elective treatments with long waiting times were reimbursed without any maximum amount to boost supply. A pilot project in 2019 for joint replacement operations focussed on optimising internal processes at the organisational level to increase the volume of activities.

Waiting times for elective surgery in **Costa Rica** have been reduced in recent years, but they remain quite long, with waits averaging about one year in 2018 for a set of surgical procedures. A new 2019-20 National Plan is designed to reduce further these waiting times (Box 4.2).

Box 4.2. Costa Rica's new 2019-20 National Plan for Timely Medical Attention of Patients on Waiting Lists

The 2019-20 National Plan for the Timely Medical Attention of Patients in Waiting Lists in Costa Rica aims to further reduce waiting times for outpatient care and elective surgery, with the project "Timely Care Plan for People" targeting patients referred for the first time to specialised medical centres. The supply of elective surgery has been increased through evening surgery and improved operating room time, and consideration is also given to introducing evening consultations with specialists. To improve efficiency, special interregional and national projects have been launched, such as the Integrated Networks for the Provision of Health Services in collaboration with national and specialised hospitals, with patients being redirected to providers with available capacity. Specific initiatives target hip and knee replacement, and cataract surgery (e.g. through the Sight Care Plan introduced in 2017), also through networks of national and regional hospitals that have started to carry out evening surgery.

The supply-side policies covered in this section are consistent with past experience in different countries showing that, in general, temporary increases of dedicated funding will only have temporary effects, and are unlikely to be successful in achieving lasting reductions in waiting times (Siciliani, Borowitz and Moran, 2013[1]). Instead, as discussed above, they can be successful if increases in resources and activities are maintained over time and if they are linked with maximum waiting times targets or guarantees, so that there are consequences for providers if progress towards meeting the maximum waiting times has not been achieved.

4.1.4. Prioritising patients on the list can contribute to reducing waiting times or the burden from waiting across patients as shown in New Zealand, Norway and Australia

Several countries have implemented prioritisation policies as a demand-side intervention to improve the management of elective surgery. Prioritisation can take two forms. First, some countries (e.g. New Zealand) have introduced policies that manage the demand by prioritising patients with different clinical needs, with the aim of avoiding to add patients on the list when the expected benefits from treatment are small or almost nil. Second, other countries (e.g. Norway, Australia and New Zealand also) have improved the prioritisation of the waiting list by re-allocating waiting times across patients and ensuring that patients with more severe conditions wait less than those lower level of severity, or by establishing different maximum waiting times for different types of patients, though the approaches can be very different across these countries.

New Zealand is a prime example of a country that has tried to improve the prioritisation of patients, though over time this demand management policy has been complemented by supply-side interventions. Since 2000, New Zealand has a national strategy for reducing waiting times for elective (or planned) care, with some amendments made in 2012. The strategy has four main objectives: i) a maximum waiting time of 6 months for a first specialist assessment (reduced to 4 months in 2012); ii) all patients with a level of need which can be met within the resources (funding) available are provided with surgery within 6 months following specialist assessment (also reduced to 4 months in 2012); iii) the delivery of a volume of publicly-funded services which is sufficient to ensure timely access to elective surgery before patients reach a state of unreasonable distress, ill health and/or incapacity; and iv) national equity of access to elective care, so that patients have similar access regardless of where they live.

The New Zealand approach is original in terms of explicitly acknowledging that the level of needs which can be met depends on available resources, therefore putting emphasis on demand management and the development and implementation of consistent clinical assessment to reduce uncertainties in the duration of the wait for patients. Clinical assessment of needs has been facilitated through the development of clinical prioritisation assessment criteria (CPAC) tools, which are multi-dimensional and integrate both objective criteria and subjective assessment. However, there are also supply elements in the policy through increasing public hospital capacity and activities.

Following the reduction in waiting times for elective surgery to a maximum of 4 months in 2012, waiting times have declined for many common elective surgical procedures (Figure 4.18) and are well below OECD averages (Figure 2.3). This reduction has been achieved through a combination of demand-side interventions as well as supply-side measures. Figure 4.19 shows that while there has been some increases in the volumes of surgical activities since in 2012, this hasn't been a sharp rise.

Figure 4.18. Waiting times for many elective surgery have decreased in New Zealand since 2012

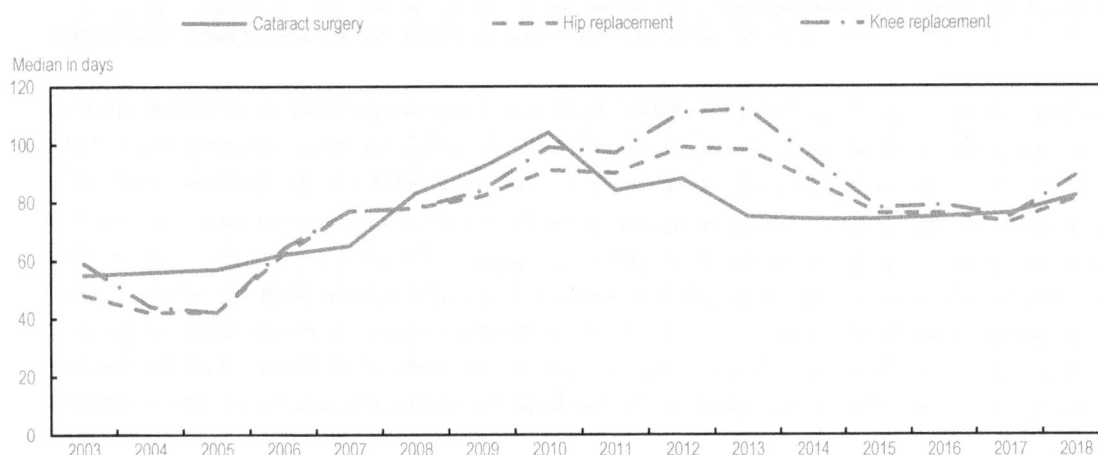

Source: OECD Health Statistics.

Figure 4.19. Increases in surgical activity rates have contributed partly to the reduction in waiting times for elective surgery in New Zealand since 2012

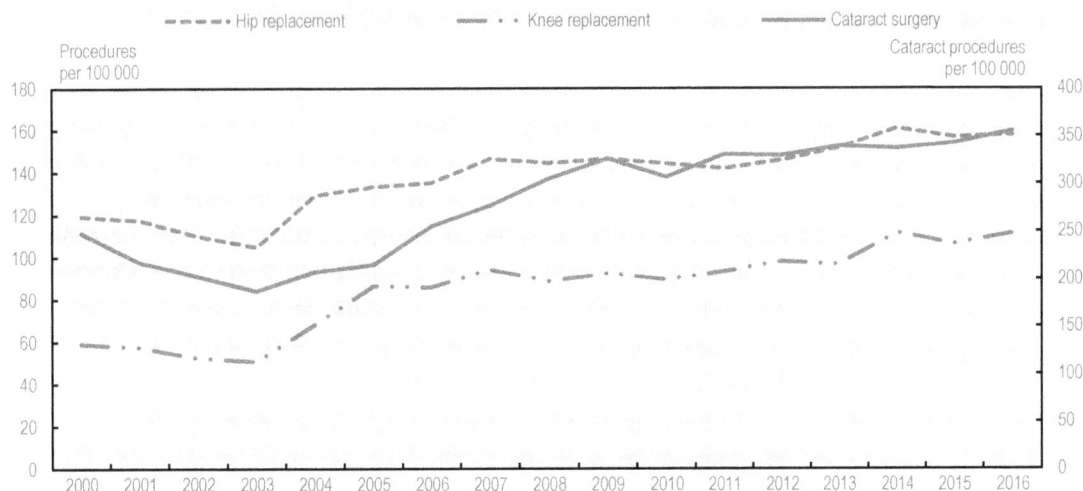

Source: OECD Health Statistics.

In 2019, the New Zealand Ministry of Health released the 'Planned Care Strategic Approach 2019-2024' to District Health Boards, which suggests a broader approach with a focus on the whole patient pathway, including also diagnostics tests. The plan is based on the principles of equity, quality, timeliness, access, and experience, and includes the following strategic priorities: balancing national consistency and local context, simplified pathways for service users, optimising sector capacity and capability, and being "fit for the future". This Strategic Approach was launched in July 2019 and is in the process of being implemented across New Zealand.

Norway has introduced, since 2002, what can be described as an individual (patient-specific) maximum waiting time guarantee that is based on the patient health condition, need and severity. This policy is still in place today. All patients who have been given a right to hospital care (as well as specialised mental health services or specialised substance abuse treatments) are assigned an individual clinically assessed maximum waiting time. This policy was motivated by the concern that maximum waiting time guarantees may cause mis-prioritisation of patients (with more complex patients waiting longer) unless this was accompanied by a clinical prioritisation. In addition, all patients have free choice of providers, both among public and certain private providers. Information about expected waiting times is published on the website where patients receive information about provider choice. This can contribute to relieve pressures on providers with capacity issues while helping providers with available capacity to maximise the use of their resources. In 2018, 98% of all patients received health care within their individual maximum waiting time.

Australia also prioritises patients based on needs, but the system is based on a simpler classification than in Norway. It involves setting waiting times for patients based on three urgency categories: Category 1 – Admission within 30 days for a condition that has the potential to deteriorate quickly to the point that it may become an emergency; Category 2 – Admission within 90 days desirable for a condition causing some pain, dysfunction or disability but is not likely to deteriorate quickly or become an emergency; and Category 3 – Admission within 365 days for a condition causing minimal or no pain, dysfunction or disability, which is unlikely to deteriorate quickly and which does not have the potential to become an emergency.

4.1.5. Several countries seek to improve the coordination between primary and secondary care to reduce waiting times for specialist consultations

Several countries have emphasised the need for better coordination between primary and second care, to ensure that referrals from primary care are appropriate and addressed in a timely manner. In **Poland**, there are plans to strengthen the role of GPs to reduce the need for ambulatory specialist care, for example by GPs expanding their role for ophthalmology and dermatology consultations, but there is a recognition that this will require additional financial incentives. In **Finland**, there are plans to increase specialist consultations taking place in primary health care centres to reduce unnecessary referrals to hospital care, in particular for patient with chronic conditions. In **Italy**, a classification system called the Homogenous Waiting Times Group has been introduced to facilitate the coordination between primary and secondary care, and ensure that both GPs and specialists assess the need and urgency in the same way and agree on assigning different maximum waiting times based on urgency with common criteria. In **Slovenia**, the pilot project on "Better management of excessive waiting times" also refers to the need of fostering better cooperation between primary and secondary care for referrals. In **Costa Rica**, there are initiatives to strengthen the appropriateness of primary care referrals for specialist care, and to introduce protocols and prioritisation criteria for referrals and diagnostics.

In **Canada**, there is no national policy on specialist visits. However, teams of health care providers from various provinces have partnered with the Canadian Foundation for Healthcare Improvement (CFHI) to spread two innovations aimed at improving coordination between primary care providers and specialists. The two innovations were the Champlain BASE™eConsult Service, a secure web-based eConsult service originally launched in the province of Ontario and the Rapid Access to Consultative Expertise (RACE™), a telephone advice line originally launched at Providence Health Care and Vancouver Coastal Health in the province of Ontario and British Columbia. The two innovations resulted in 4 in 5 eConsults receiving a response from a specialist within 7 days. More than half (53%) of eConsults avoided any face-to-face referral to a specialist, while 40% of eConsults avoided an emergency department visit.

Digital consultations are becoming increasingly common since the COVID-19 pandemic to limit physical contacts, and a growing number of countries have either introduced or extended the possibilities of teleconsultations (OECD, 2020[34]).

4.2. Policies to reduce waiting times for primary care

In many OECD countries, primary care delivered by general practitioners (GPs) is the first level of contact for the population with the health care system. Timely access to high-quality primary care is crucial to improve health, reduce inequalities, and make the health system more efficient (OECD, 2020[35]). Half the countries that responded to the OECD questionnaire consider waiting times in primary care an issue (Figure 1.3).

4.2.1. Maximum waiting time targets in primary care generally range between 1 and 7 days

Some countries – primarily in Northern Europe but also some regions in Spain – have set maximum waiting times for primary care (Table 4.2). The Baltic countries (Estonia, Latvia and Lithuania) all require urgent patients to be seen within one day, while non-urgent cases should be seen within 5 to 7 days. Norway and Iceland require a consultation within 5 or 6 days, respectively[5]. In Spain, maximum waiting times are set at the regional level, and vary from 1 to 3 days in those regions that have set such a maximum. In Finland, all patients should be seen on the day when they contact a primary care centre and a further evaluation of their care needs (if needed) should take place within 3 days.

Table 4.2. Maximum waiting times for primary care

Country	Maximum waiting times
Estonia	• In case of an urgent health problem, patients should be able contact/visit to their GP's on same day. • In case of non-acute health problem within 5 working days.
Finland	• Same day • Further evaluation of need for care within 3 days
Iceland	• GP consultation/visit within 6 days
Latvia	• GP for acute patients: 1 working day • GP consultations/visit for non-acute patients: 5 working days
Lithuania	• Primary care for acute patients: 24hours • Primary care for non-acute patients: 7 calendar days
Norway	• Appointment normally within 5 days
Spain	Pais Vasco • 3 days Baleares • 2 days Madrid • same day/without delay

Source: OECD Waiting Times questionnaire 2019.

4.2.2. Supply-side policies focus on expanding the primary care workforce and extending opening hours

The number of (GPs) per population varies widely across OECD countries, although some of the variation is due to differences in the ways doctors are categorised across countries. For example, in the United States, general internal medicine doctors often play a role similar to that of GPs (family doctors) in other countries, yet they are categorised as specialists. On average across OECD countries, there were 0.77 GPs per 1 000 population in 2017 (or about 1 300 population for every GP), but this number was much lower in some countries (Figure 4.20). In most countries, the number of GPs as a share of all doctors has decreased over the past two decades.

Figure 4.20. The number of GPs is very low in some OECD countries, 2017 (or nearest year)

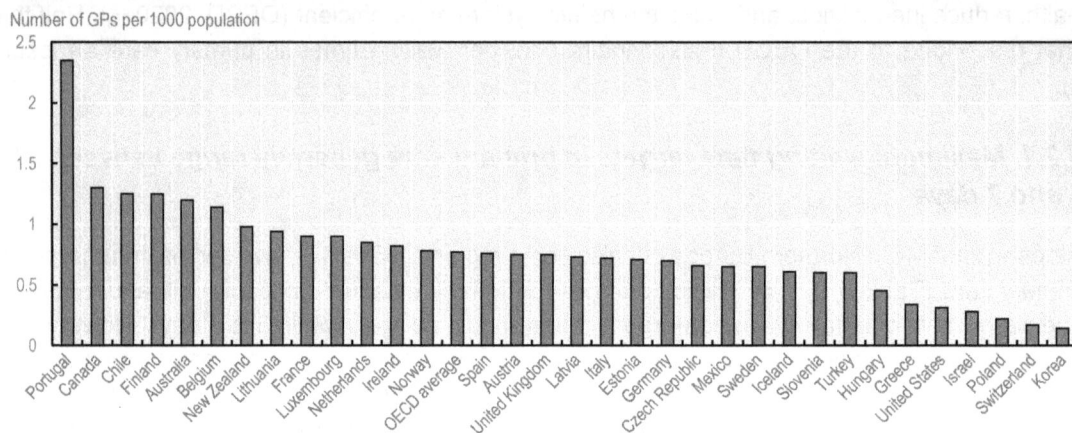

Number of GPs per 1000 population

Note: The number of GPs in Portugal, Chile and Greece is over-estimated as it includes all doctors licensed to practice, not only those actually practising. In the United States and other countries, GPs do not include general internal medicine doctors (who are categorised as specialists) although they often play a role similar to that of GPs.
Source: OECD Health Statistics.

Several countries have taken initiatives to increase the availability of primary care physicians. In Norway, municipalities are working to recruit and retain GPs in response to increasing demand for services. Luxembourg has developed a specific training in general medical practice at the University of Luxembourg. Portugal has significantly increased the training of family doctors and the recruitment of physicians for the NHS primary care units in recent years. Costa Rica is increasing the number of EBAIS (Basic Teams for Comprehensive Health Care), which are located in communities across the country, as well as the number of specialists in Family Medicine, to reduce waiting times for primary care.

Lithuania has implemented the Family Medicine Development Action Plan for 2016-2025, which aims to increase the number of family doctors and ensure their adequate distribution – amongst other objectives. Lithuania also expanded the family doctor team with nurse assistants, social services workers, lifestyle medical specialists and physiotherapists. These professionals can provide effective, high-quality services while lowering the workload for GPs. In 2019, Lithuania expanded the clinical competencies of general practice nurses, allowing them to coordinate the tasks of nurse assistants, prescribe medicinal products in some situations, monitor the progression of chronic diseases, prescribe routine urine and blood tests, and interpret their results.

Many other countries have expanded the role of different primary care providers beyond GPs to improve timely access while maintaining a role of leaders for GPs in primary care teams. Many countries have reported that nurses or physician assistants can deliver a growing number of services in primary care, including providing immunisation, health education and routine checks of patients with chronic conditions (Table 4.3). For example, since 2010, family nurses in Estonia can give consultations and counselling to certain groups, including patients with chronic diseases, pregnant women and healthy neonates. Cooperation between solo practices in rural areas and the creation of group practices has also been incentivised by the government, to help cover holidays and unexpected sick leave.

In the United Kingdom, the 2019 GP five-year contract framework provides funding to 20 000 non-GP roles in general practice, including pharmacists, physician associates and first contact physiotherapists. These roles have been chosen as they can reduce GP workload (NHS, 2019[36]).

Table 4.3. Involvement of nurses or physician assistants in health promotion and prevention, 2016

	At least 75% of nurses or physician assistants can provide immunisations	At least 75% of nurses or physician assistants can provide health education	At least 75% of nurses or physician assistants can provide routine checks of chronically ill patients
Austria	No	No	No
Belgium	No	No	No
Canada	No	Yes	Yes
Chile	Yes	Yes	Yes
Czech Republic	Yes	No	No
Denmark	No	Yes	No
Estonia	Yes	Yes	Yes
Finland	Yes	Yes	Yes
France	No	Yes	No
Greece	No	Yes	Yes
Iceland	Yes	No	No
Ireland	Yes	Yes	Yes
Israel	Yes	Yes	Yes
Italy	No	No	No
Latvia	Yes	Yes	Yes
Luxembourg	No	No	No
Netherlands	Yes	Yes	Yes
Norway	No	No	No
Poland	Yes	Yes	Yes
Portugal	Yes	Yes	Yes
Slovenia	No	No	No
Spain	Yes	Yes	Yes
Sweden	Yes	Yes	Yes
Switzerland	No	Yes	No
Turkey	Yes	NR	NR
United Kingdom	Yes	Yes	Yes
Total "yes" responses (out of 26 countries)	15	17	14

Source: OECD (2016[37]), Health System Characteristics Survey, http://www.oecd.org/els/health-systems/characteristics.htm.

In many OECD countries, seeing a GP outside normal working hours is difficult for a substantial proportion of the population, often resulting in visits to hospital emergency departments. The survey on the quality and costs of primary care (QUALICOPC) carried out in 2013 showed that over 30% of the population in a dozen of countries reported then that it was too difficult to see a GP during evenings, nights and weekends (Figure 4.21). Many countries have taken steps to increase access to care outside of normal operating hours and in doing so reduce the waiting times for primary care.

Figure 4.21. In many countries, general practitioners are not available outside normal hours, 2013

% of patients reporting difficulties seeing GPs outside normal working hours

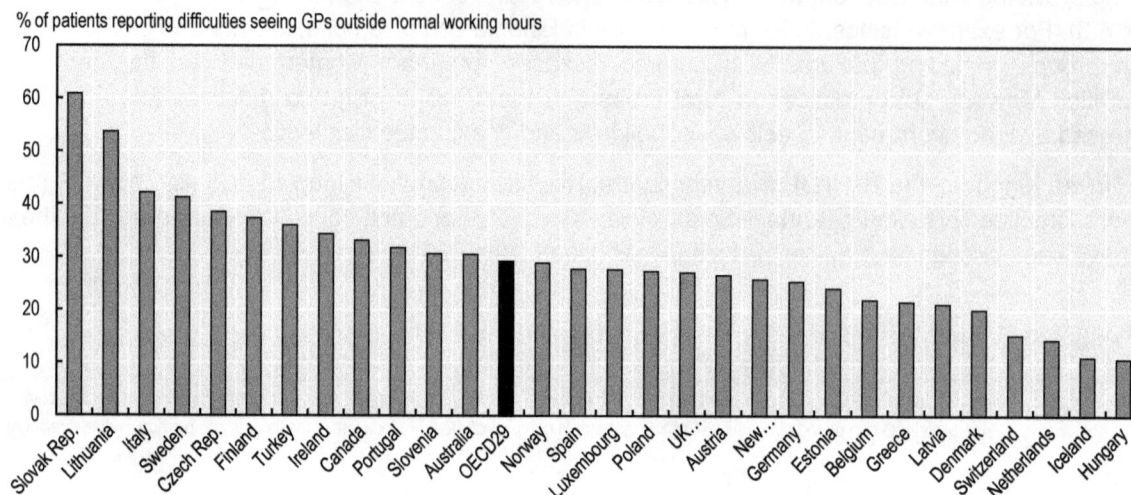

Source: OECD estimates based on QUALICOPC (2013).

A more recent survey led by the Commonwealth Fund found that the proportion of primary care practices that had arrangements in place for patients to be seen when they are closed exceeded 90% in Germany, New Zealand, Norway and the Netherlands in 2019, while less than half of primary care practices in the United States and Canada had these arrangements in place (Figure 4.22).

Figure 4.22. Less than half of primary care practices in the United States and Canada have arrangements in place where patients can be seen when the practice is closed

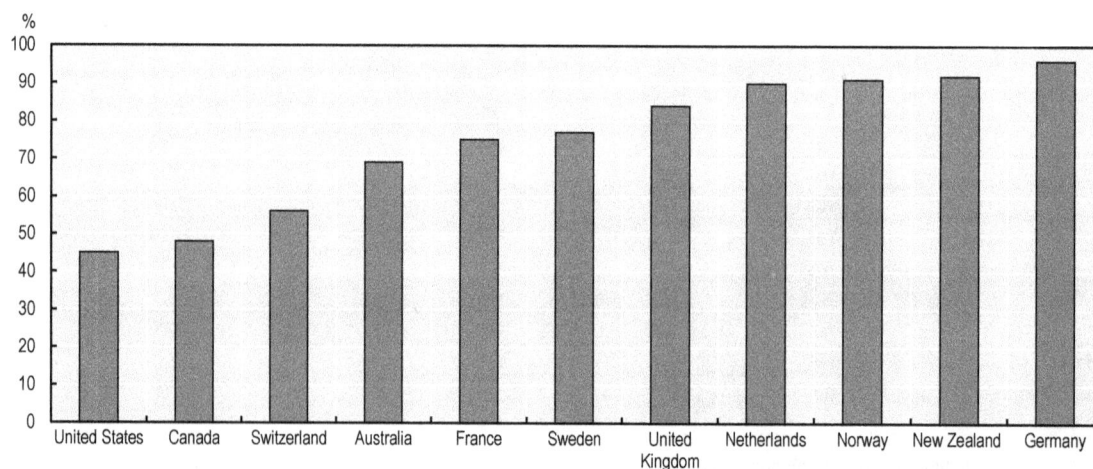

Source: 2019 Commonwealth Fund International Health Policy Survey of Primary Care Physicians.

Australia has financial incentives for primary care practices to provide timely care, under the Practice Incentive Program (PIP). The PIP After Hours Incentive encourages practices to provide patients with access to quality after-hours GP care. In Luxembourg, the Ministry of Health funds "Maisons Médicale de garde" (medical on-call centres) to provide out-of-hours primary care.

4.2.1. New technologies are used to increase access and reduce waiting times on both the demand and supply side

While the use of telemedicine in OECD countries was quite limited before the COVID-19 crisis (Oliveira Hashiguchi, 2020[38]), some countries had already turned to new technologies to increase the supply of primary care services. Australia had already developed new payment models to fund the provision of teleconsultations, and access to teleconsultations have been accelerated and broadened in March 2020 to reduce the spread of COVID-19. Since 2013, teleconsultations have also been covered under the Estonian Health Insurance Fund, as well as e-referrals to improve coordination between primary and secondary care. These teleconsultations are likely to become even more prominent in the future, in particular for the elderly and people with chronic conditions to reduce their risk of catching serious infectious diseases like COVID-19 (OECD, 2020[34]).

Digital technology has also been used to address the demand side of waiting times. Luxembourg has developed a mobile phone app called "DispoDoc" in collaboration with the e-Health Agency and the Society of General Practitioners. The app shows the GP practices that are open in the immediate surroundings of the patient, including outside of usual opening hours. In Mexico, some institutions are using appointment scheduling via internet that takes into account the number of doctors available in the different departments, to minimise the waiting times. Australians can access health information and advice via Health Direct, a free 24 hour help line. It is staffed by registered nurses who provide a triage service and access to an after-hours GP helpline. In areas where there are no GPs, Health Direct provides a call-back service from a GP who can provide advice over the phone.

4.3. Policies to reduce waiting times for cancer care

Waiting times for cancer care is considered to be an issue in the majority of OECD countries (Figure 1.3), but not in some countries like the Czech Republic, Iceland, Ireland, Israel, Japan, the Netherlands and Slovenia. However, in some of the countries where waiting time is not considered to be an issue, waiting times for cancer care are relatively long. For example, in Iceland, about 20% of patients in early 2019 had been waiting for more than 3 months for a breast cancer surgery.

In Canada and the United Kingdom, waiting time strategies have been developed to reduce waiting times for cancer care as part of broader waiting time policies. In Canada, federal, provincial and territorial governments committed in 2004 to reduce waiting times in cancer care and to improve waiting time data reporting. The United Kingdom involves a wide range of stakeholders (including health professional bodies and patient groups) in developing operational standards for waiting times in cancer care.

Several OECD countries (e.g. Denmark, Ireland, Latvia, Lithuania and New Zealand) aim to ensure timely access to cancer care under the national cancer control programme. For example, Lithuania has introduced a National Cancer Prevention and Control Programme for the period 2014-2025, with one of the main objectives being to improve timely access to diagnostic services and treatment for cancer patients. The New Zealand Government is developing a ten-year Cancer Action Plan for the period 2019-2029, which will aim to improve services across all cancer control activities including waiting times for diagnosis and treatment.

4.3.1. To tackle long waiting times in cancer care, the majority of OECD countries set waiting time targets and regularly evaluate the progress

OECD countries have implemented a range of policy measures to tackle waiting times for cancer care, including: 1) the introduction of maximum waiting time targets; 2) the regular evaluation and assessment of waiting times; 3) the introduction of fast track pathway; 4) the provision of financial support to increase the capacity and delivery of cancer care; and 5) a reorganisation of cancer care delivery and efforts to improve care coordination. About half of OECD countries set waiting time targets, which is accompanied by regular monitoring of progress in meeting these waiting time targets (Table 4.4).

Table 4.4. Policy measures taken to reduce waiting time for cancer care

Policy options	Waiting time targets	Regular evaluation/assessment of waiting times	Fast track pathway	Financial support to increase capacity and delivery of cancer care	Reorganisation of cancer care delivery and improving care coordination
Countries	Canada, Costa Rica, Denmark, Estonia, Finland, Hungary, Iceland, Ireland, Latvia, Lithuania, Luxembourg, New Zealand, Norway, Portugal, Slovenia, Spain (some regions), United Kingdom	Canada, Costa Rica, Denmark, Estonia, Finland, Hungary, Iceland, Ireland, Latvia, Lithuania, Luxembourg, New Zealand, Norway, Poland, Portugal, Slovak Republic, Slovenia, Spain (some regions), United Kingdom	Denmark, Ireland, Latvia, Poland, Slovenia, Spain (some regions)	Australia, Hungary, Latvia, Poland, Slovenia, Slovak Republic	Finland, Greece, Japan, Luxembourg, Netherlands, Slovenia

Source: OECD Waiting Time Project Policy Questionnaire 2019 and OECD (2013[39]).

4.3.2. Maximum waiting time targets for cancer care

Many OECD countries set maximum waiting times for cancer care that vary according to services and clinical assessment of urgency of diagnosis and treatment (Table 4.5).

There are variations in maximum waiting times for the same service across countries. For instance, while Hungary set waiting time targets of 2 weeks for CT and MRI scan in suspected cases of cancer, the maximum waiting time set for such diagnostic tests in Lithuania is two-times longer (4 weeks). In Estonia, the maximum waiting time for specialist care is 8 months for all patients including cancer patients.

Table 4.5. Maximum waiting times for cancer care

Country	Maximum waiting times
Canada	Waiting time for radiotherapy treatment – 28 days
Costa Rica	Average waiting period <90 days
Denmark	Waiting time between the receipt of referral from doctor to the notification by hospital on the possibility of providing treatment within maximum waiting time by hospital – 11 calendar days
Estonia	Outpatient consultation/visit maximum length of waiting time – 6 weeks Specialist care (inpatient and day care) maximum length of waiting time – 8 months Planned home nursing care for cancer patients: 2 weeks
Finland	Interval between the arrival of a referral concerning a suspected case of cancer and the start of the primary treatment – 6 weeks Interval between surgical treatment and adjuvant therapies – 4 weeks although depending on the patient's state of health
Hungary	Cancer diagnostics (CT and MRI scan): 2 weeks
Iceland	Time between a decision-to-treat and first cancer treatment – 31 days Time between a referral with a highly suspected case of cancer and first cancer treatment – 62 days
Ireland	Time between the receipt of referral and an appointment for patients with breast cancer symptoms, meeting clinical criteria for urgent referral to a symptomatic breast disease clinic – 2 weeks (target 95% of patients) Time between the receipt of referral and an appointment for patients with breast cancer symptoms, meeting clinical criteria for non-urgent referral to a symptomatic breast disease clinic – 12 weeks (target 95% of patients) Time between the receipt of referral and an appointment at Rapid Access Clinic for patients with suspected lung cancer – 10 working days (target 95% of patients) Time between the receipt of referral and an appointment at Rapid Access Clinic for men with suspected prostate cancer – 20 working days (target 90% of patients)

Country	Maximum waiting times
Latvia	Waiting time for examinations after screening programme – 30 days Waiting time for primary diagnostic test of malignant tumours from the date of referral by a family doctor or gynaecologist – 10 working days Waiting time for specialists visit for secondary diagnosis of malignant tumours after oncological consultation following primary diagnostics – 10 working days Waiting time for treatment strategies for patient (surgery, chemotherapy, radiotherapy) after secondary diagnosis of malignant – 1 month
Lithuania	Waiting time between the first visit to specialist to the date of cancer diagnosis – 28 calendar days Waiting time from the registration to get expensive diagnostic test (CT and/or MRI and/or PET) to the date when the diagnostic test was performed – 30 calendar days Waiting time from the registration date to receive chemotherapy, radiotherapy, haematology services to the date when services were received – 30 calendar days Waiting time from the registration to get surgery to the date of the operation – 60 calendar days
Luxembourg	Diagnosis within 5 working days for at least 95% of patients Guidelines of patient pathways from the National Cancer Institute of Luxembourg have been published with specific targets for patients affected by prostate cancer, breast cancer, lung cancer and colorectal cancer (e.g. time between chemotherapy and radiotherapy is maximum 4 weeks, or 2 weeks after the analytical report has been received)
New Zealand	Decision-to-treat to first treatment: 31 days Referral with high suspicion of cancer to first treatment: 62 days
Norway	Standardised waiting times based on the condition
Portugal	Priority level 4 : 72 hours Priority level 3 : 15 days Priority level 2 : 45 days Priority level 1 (normal): 60 days
Spain	Aragon, Baleares, Cantabria, Madrid, Navarra: 30 days until surgery
United Kingdom	93% of patients to have a maximum two week wait from GP referral for urgent referrals where cancer is suspected 96% of patients to have maximum one month (31-day) wait from diagnosis to first definitive treatment for all cancers 85% of patients to have a maximum two month (62-day) wait from urgent referral for suspected cancer to first treatment for all cancers 93% of patients to have a maximum two week wait to see a specialist for all patients referred for investigation of breast symptoms, even if cancer is not initially suspected 94% of patients to have a maximum 31-day wait for subsequent treatment where the treatment is surgery 94% of patients to have a maximum 31-day wait for subsequent treatment where the treatment is a course of radiotherapy 98% of patients to have a maximum 31-day wait for subsequent treatment where the treatment is an anti-cancer drug regiment 90% of patients to have a maximum 62-day wait from referral from an NHS cancer screening service to first definitive treatment for cancer.

Note: This table includes only waiting time targets specific to cancer care pathways; it excludes general targets for diagnostic or elective procedures that may also apply to cancer care.
Source: OECD Waiting Times Policy Questionnaire 2019.

4.3.3. Regular evaluation and assessment of waiting times for cancer care

In all OECD countries where waiting time targets for cancer care have been developed, waiting times are regularly monitored and assessed (Table 4.5). For instance, Denmark established integrated patient pathways for cancer patients and monitors pathway of cancer patients from whether they are examined and/or treated within recommended time periods. These data are monitored quarterly and annually and disaggregated by cancer and region. In 2015, Norway introduced standardised patient pathways covering diagnosis, treatment and rehabilitation for different cancers, and monitors whether targets are achieved within patient pathways specific to 26 cancers every four months and annually. In Iceland, the number of people on the waiting lists and the percentage of people waiting more than three months among all the people on the waiting lists are reported every three months by hospital or clinic for specific procedures related to cancer care. Latvia also monitors and reports each year waiting times for certain cancer care, such as colonoscopy, mammography, chemotherapy and radiation therapy in day care, and oncologist by medical institution.

Greece and Mexico are the only two countries that consider waiting times to be an issue for cancer care, but have not yet conducted any regular monitoring and assessment.

Regular monitoring of waiting times for cancer care has been accompanied by progress in reducing waiting times in some countries, but progress in other countries has been mixed or limited. In Estonia, for example, the average number of days that patients wait to get an appointment with an oncologist has been cut down by nearly half between 2008 and 2018 (from 15 days to 8 days), yet the proportion of patients who had to wait at least 6 weeks to get a consultation with an oncologist has increased in recent years, indicating that many patients are waiting longer.

In many OECD countries, waiting times for cancer care have been stable over time and in some cases such as in Canada, Ireland, Spain (Aragon) and the United Kingdom, meeting maximum waiting time targets for some cancer services have become more difficult in recent years (Figure 4.23). In the United Kingdom, while the proportion of patients who receive their first treatment within 31 days of a decision to treat has remained stable and above the standard (or target) of 96% in recent years, the proportion of patients who receive their first treatment within 62 days of an urgent GP referral has fallen below the standard of 85% to 79% in 2018. This is partly because the proportion of people who saw a specialist within 2 weeks of an urgent GP referral also fell below the standard of 93% (Figure 4.24).

Figure 4.23. The proportion of cancer patients waiting more than 30 days increased in recent years in Spain (Aragon)

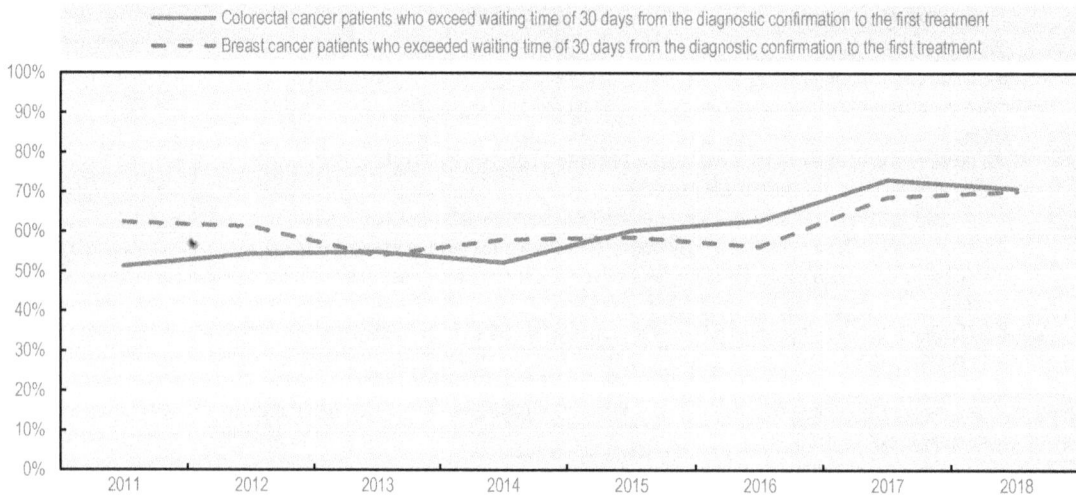

Source: OECD Waiting Time Data Questionnaire 2019.

Figure 4.24. Some waiting time standards for cancer care have not been met in recent years in the United Kingdom

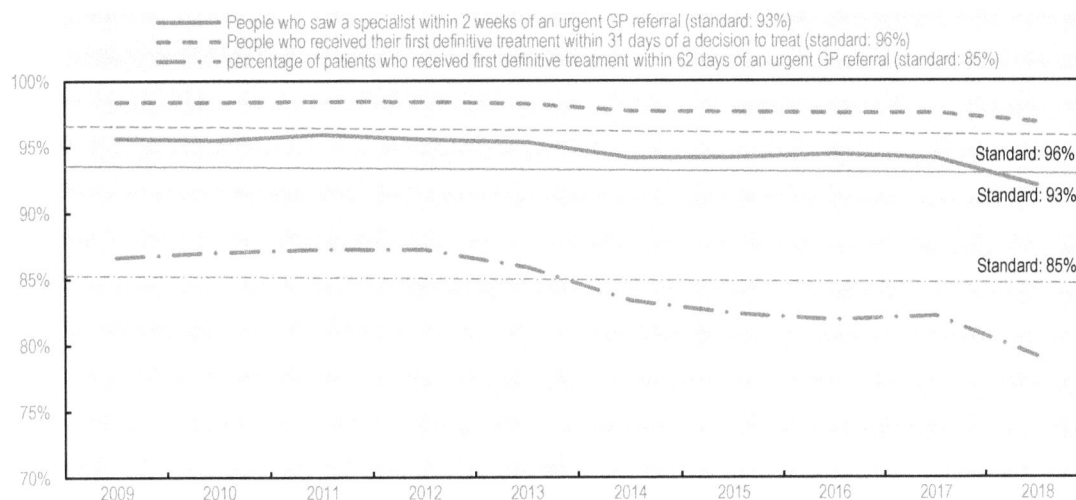

Source: OECD Waiting Time Data Questionnaire 2019.

4.3.4. Fast track pathway for cancer patients

Many countries (e.g. Denmark, Ireland, Latvia, Poland, Slovenia and some regions in Spain) introduced a fast track to diagnose and treat cancer patients. In Poland, for example, under the Rapid Oncology Therapy package introduced in 2015, if suspected cancer is confirmed, a doctor issues a Cancer Diagnosis and Treatment Card (DiLO Card), which allows fast track treatment. Latvia also introduced fast track access for cancer patients (called Green Corridor/Tunnel) in 2016. The proportion of cancer patients diagnosed at early stages has increased from 50% in 2015 to 55% in 2017. The longest waiting time for a mammography, chemotherapy and radiation therapy has also decreased by 4 days, 54 days and 10 days respectively between 2015 and 2019 (to reach 28 days, 42 days and 32 days). However, during the same period, the longest waiting time has increased to get a colonoscopy from 82 to 144 days. Although the average waiting times to get an appointment with an oncologist across has decreased between 2013 and 2019, waiting times in some institutions are still very long (Figure 4.25).

Figure 4.25. Waiting time for oncologist in Latvia has become shorter in most hospital and clinics providing cancer care in 2019 compared to 2013, but the longest waiting time has become longer

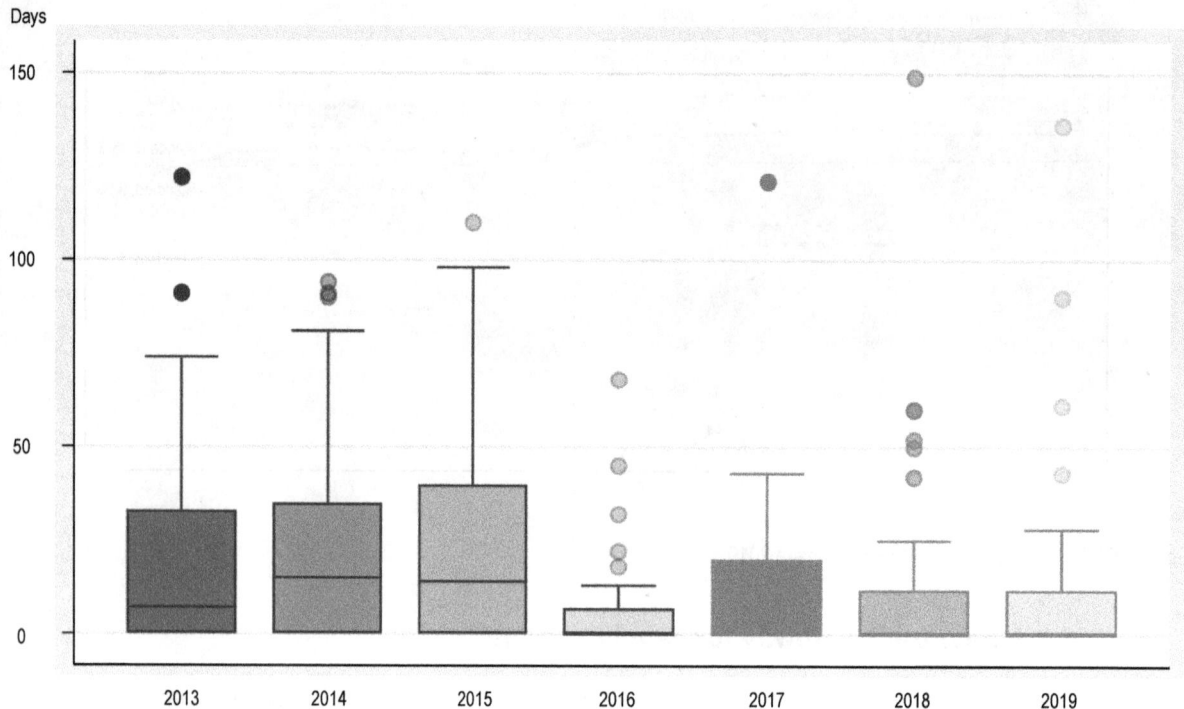

Note: Data refer to the waiting time for oncologist in each medical institution with an oncologist during the month of February. The box shows up to the 75th percentiles while the bar in the box refers to the median. The H shows an upper value (75th percentile plus 1.5 times the difference between the 75th percentile and 25th percentile) while the dots show the outliers.
Source: OECD Waiting Time Data Questionnaire 2019.

4.3.5. Financial support to increase capacity and delivery for cancer care

Several OECD countries have increased funding to expand the capacity to deliver cancer care more rapidly. This has been the case notably in several Central and Eastern European countries (Hungary, Latvia, Poland and Slovenia) where the resources allocated to cancer care were historically more limited. Poland provides financial support to realise timely provision of cancer care under the Rapid Oncology Therapy package. Similarly, in Latvia, services provided under the Green Corridor/Tunnel (fast track) have been financed fully by the state budget.

In Australia, the variation in access to radiotherapy across states as well as between rural and urban areas has been addressed through regular additional investment in equipment and trained staff to deal with insufficient resources, with success in reducing such geographic inequality (OECD, 2013[39]).

However, as is the case for other elective treatment, increasing the supply of resources and treatments for different types of cancer provides no guarantee that waiting times will fall if the demand also increases. In Ireland, for instance, breast cancer surgery has increased between 2010 and 2018, particularly the number of total mastectomy which has grown by nearly 20%. Nonetheless, during this period, the proportion of patients who underwent surgical intervention within 20 working days of the date of multidisciplinary team meeting has decreased from 90% to 76% (Figure 4.26).

Figure 4.26. Even though breast cancer surgery increased, the proportion of patients treated within less than 20 working days has decreased in Ireland since 2010

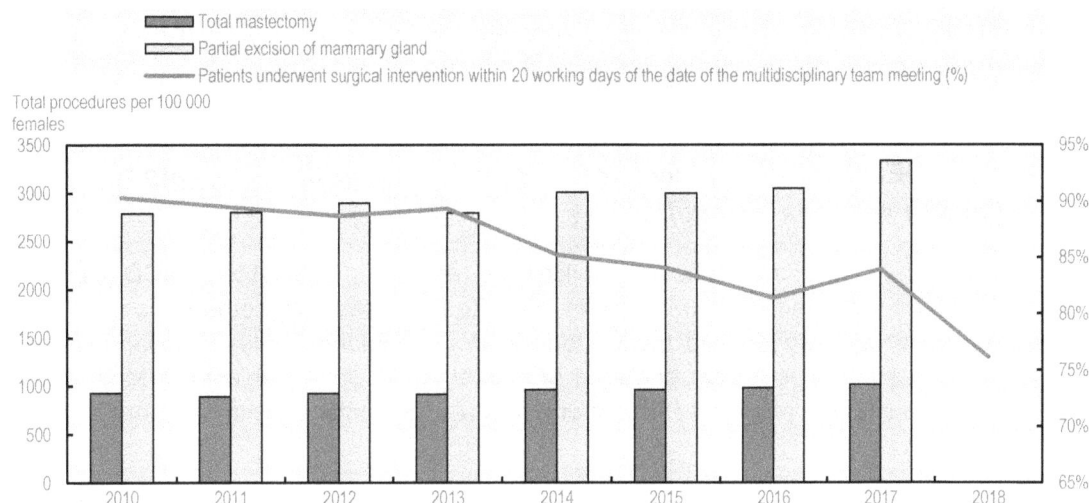

Source: OECD Health Statistics 2019 and OECD Waiting Time Data Questionnaire 2019.

4.3.6. Reorganisation of cancer care delivery and promotion of greater care coordination

Some OECD countries (e.g. Finland and Luxembourg) have undertaken a reorganisation of cancer care delivery to improve the quality of cancer care and reduce waiting times. In order to resolve waiting times for diagnosis of cancer, since 2016 Luxembourg has conducted a comprehensive reorganisation of National Health Laboratory's diagnostic services by reducing outsourcing to laboratories abroad and fully operationalising the management of these services in the main hospitals. This reorganisation has resulted in eliminating waiting times longer than 14 working days for such diagnosis.

In 2016, the Ministry of Social Affairs and Health in Finland announced the establishment of a new National Cancer Centre, with a responsibility to ensure equal and timely access to cancer care and promote quality of care. It started its activities in 2018.

Norway has also launched a number of initiatives in recent years to improve access and quality of cancer care. Cancer patient pathways were introduced in 2015 for 28 different types of cancer to reduce unnecessary waiting times and improve coordination of care. Throughout the course of treatment and in the follow-up period the patient is assigned a designated pathway coordinator responsible for ensuring continuity of care.

In Slovenia, the coordination between professionals were strengthened with the introduction of a breast cancer screening programme and immediate access has been pursued for patients diagnosed through the programme, leading to a reduction of referral time in the 2000s. The colorectal cancer screening programme, introduced in 2009, also aims to shorten waiting times between screening and diagnostic colonoscopy and between colonoscopy and first treatment. In Italy, in some regions, particularly in the north, a disease management programme has introduced a scheduled follow-up, providing timely cancer care through organised care coordination. Denmark introduced National Integrated Pathways in 2007 to reduce delays, and implemented them for all cancer diagnosis in 2008 (OECD, 2013[39]).

4.4. Policies to reduce waiting times for mental health care

In OECD countries, between one in five and one in six people are living with a mental illness at any time (OECD/European Union, 2018[40]). Timely access to services can help people recover from a mental illness, or help them to manage the symptoms and reduce the impact on their lives. At least ten OECD countries have maximum waiting times targets for mental health services.

4.4.1. Many OECD countries have set maximum waiting times targets for mental health services for adults

Waiting times targets in the area of mental health services are reported in at least ten OECD countries. Denmark, Finland, Ireland, Lithuania, the Netherlands, New Zealand, Norway, some regions in Spain (including Baleares, Navarra), Sweden and the United Kingdom (England, Wales, Scotland) have a waiting times target or guarantee in at least one area of mental health care (Table 4.6).[6] Most waiting times targets or guarantees aim to provide treatment or a first service contact within 1-3 months.

Table 4.6. Maximum waiting times for mental health services

Country	Maximum waiting times
Denmark	• Extended free hospital choice means you have the right to receive examination or treatment in a private hospital if you have to wait more than 30 days
Finland	• Young people up to 23 years: 3 months • Referred patient assessed by a specialist in 3 weeks. • Treatment in 3 months (may be extended to 6 months for less urgent cases)
Ireland	• 90% of accepted referrals / re-referrals offered first appointment within 12 weeks by General Adult Community Mental Health Team • 75% of accepted referrals / re-referrals offered first appointment and seen within 12 weeks by General Adult Community Mental Health Team
Lithuania	• Primary mental health care: 7 calendar days • Specialist mental health care: 30 calendar days
Netherlands	• Time to referral: 4 weeks • From referral to treatment: 10 weeks • Total waiting time to treatment: 14 weeks
New Zealand	• 80% of new child and youth clients seen by specialist mental health and addiction services within 3 weeks • 95% of new child and youth clients seen by specialist mental health and addiction services within 8 weeks
Norway	• % of patients who have received health care within the clinically assessed deadline assigned to the patient • Target: average for adults: 45 days (40 in 2020) • Target: average for children under 18: 40 days (35 in 2020) Substance abuse treatment • Target: average 35 days (30 in 2020) • Guarantee for children and youth below 23 years with mental health or substance addiction: 65 days
Spain	Baleares: • Less than 60 days Navarra: • Ordinarily less than 30 business days, preferred less than 10 business days
Sweden	• After an initial examination, no patient should have to wait more than 90 days to see a specialist, and no more than 90 days for an operation or treatment, once it has been determined what care is needed • 30 days for children and adolescents (note: to be confirmed)

Country	Maximum waiting times
United Kingdom	England • 50% of people experiencing first episode psychosis commence treatment within two weeks of referral • 75% of people referred to the IAPT programme of psychological therapies begin treatment within 6 weeks of referral, and 95% begin treatment within 18 weeks Scotland • A maximum wait of 18 weeks from a patient's referral to treatment for Psychological Therapies for at least 90% of patients • A maximum wait of 18 weeks for children and young people waiting for treatment in mental health services for at least 90% of patients Wales • People referred for a mental health assessment should be seen within 28 days of receipt of referral. Following assessment there is a 28-day target to ensure people have timely access to treatment following the assessment outcome • For children and adolescents: urgent referrals within 48 hours, routine referrals within 28 days

Source: OECD Waiting Times questionnaire except for the following countries: Sweden (https://sweden.se/society/health-care-in-sweden/) England (https://www.england.nhs.uk/mentalhealth/wp-content/uploads/sites/29/2016/04/eip-guidance.pdf; https://www.england.nhs.uk/wp-content/uploads/2015/02/iapt-wait-times-guid.pdf); Scotland (https://www.isdscotland.org/Health-Topics/Waiting-Times/Waiting-Times-Statistics/); Wales (https://www.nhsdirect.wales.nhs.uk/encyclopaedia/w/article/waitingtimes/).

Since 2019, Norway has introduced standardised patient pathways within mental health services, and maximum waiting times between different points along the patient pathway have been set. Australia will track waiting times in youth mental health centres. In Canada, waiting times for mental health services are recorded at the provincial or territorial level, and efforts to introduce a national collection of waiting time indicators are ongoing.

4.4.2. Service- or condition-specific waiting times tracking or targets may offer more insights into levels of demand and access

Mental health care comprises a multitude of different conditions, severities, and service types. Some countries, for example Ireland, the Netherlands, Denmark and Finland, appear to track waiting times for all mental health care from the point of referral. Other countries, for example England, distinguish between different types of services, while the Netherlands records waiting times by category of disorder diagnosis. In the Netherlands, the average waiting time until the start of treatment varies from 12 weeks for schizophrenia and other psychotic disorders, to 18 weeks for personality disorders, while the target for waiting time is 14 weeks for all disorders (Nederlandse Zorgautoriteit, 2018[41]). In Norway, different waiting time targets are set for specialist mental health care, and specialist addiction care, while New Zealand also tracks waiting times for addiction care separately from mental health services.

For some conditions, a short waiting time can improve the therapeutic efficacy of services. Some countries have linked their waiting times targets to clinical guidelines for services or conditions, or assessments have been made of clinically acceptable wait times. There does not appear to be significant consistency between countries in terms of the waiting times targets they set, and only one country (England) distinguishes between targets set for different specialist mental health services. While it is understood that countries excluded patients needing urgent and emergency care from waiting lists, only one country (Norway) appears to differentiate waiting time target according to the individual patient's needs.

The Canadian Psychiatric Association prepared a series of waiting time benchmarks for serious psychiatric illness, published in 2006, with wait indications ranging from 2 weeks (for urgent care or first episode psychosis) to 4 weeks (for depression, and other diagnostic and management consultations) (Canadian Psychiatric Association, 2006[42]).

In England, two waiting time standards for mental health services were introduced from 2015 (NHS England, 2015[43]). The two standards with waiting times targets are for Early Intervention in Psychosis

(2 weeks from referral to treatment), and access to England's psychological therapies programme (75% of people with common mental health conditions treated within 6 weeks, 95% within 18 weeks). These standards also assess 'NICE concordance', which is the degree to which the treatment delivered at the target time meets standards for clinical best practice. All waiting times standards are established in line with evidence from England's NICE standards for evidence-based care. For example, access to Early Intervention in Psychosis services can reduce the likelihood of an individual receiving compulsory treatment from 44% to 23% during the first two months of psychosis (which is also cost saving), and reduce a young person's suicide risk from 15% to 1% (NHS England, 2015[43]; NICE, 2014[44]). For this care, timely access to appropriate services can significantly improve outcomes in the long term (NHS England, 2015[43]).

4.4.3. Several OECD countries have waiting times guarantees or targets for children and adolescents

Several countries (Finland, Ireland, New Zealand, Norway, Sweden, Scotland, Wales) report separate waiting times guarantees for mental health services for children and adolescents. Waiting time targets appear to be similar, or slightly shorter, for children and young people. For example, in Norway, the target for children and young people (40 days) is slightly shorter than for adults (45 days). In Sweden, the wait time target is much shorter for children and young people (30 days) than for adults (90 days).

New Zealand has a wait time target for children and young peoples' mental health services, but not for adult services (although wait times data is collected for adult services). Australia will start collecting waiting times information for children and adolescents, but does not do so for adults. In Australia, the "headspace" programme (a programme created in 2006 to support young people aged from 12 to 25 years to reduce the impact of depression, anxiety, stress, and alcohol and drug use) is the preferred model of youth mental health service delivery, and will be required to collect data and undertake research and analysis to regularly report on wait times across the headspace network.

In Ontario, Canada, long and growing mental health wait lists for children and adolescents are seen as a signal that mental health care availability was insufficient (Global News Canada, 2020[45]; Ipsos, 2020[46]). Between 2017 and 2020 the number of children and youth on waiting lists for mental health services doubled, from 12 000 to 28 000, with an average wait for care 67-92 days depending on the service, but the longest waits reaching 919 days or 2.5 years (Children's Mental Health Ontario, 2020[47]).

4.4.4. Maximum waiting times targets or guarantees are met for a growing proportion of people in some countries

Where data is available over time, the proportion of patients who have been assessed or treated within the maximum waiting times targets appears to have increased in many countries and average waiting times decreased for mental health care. While data is not comparable between countries as they cover different types of mental health services and maximum waiting times for these services, some countries submitted time series data for adult mental health services (Denmark, Estonia, Finland, Norway), and time series data could be found for England. Based on these data, the proportion of persons meeting the waiting time target appears to have been stable or increasing over the past five years in most countries. In Denmark, the proportion of patients assessed and investigated within 30 days increased from 91% in 2016 to 94% in 2017 and 2018. In Finland, the proportion of patients who waited less than 90 days increased from 85% in 2012, to 93% in 2018, with a brief drop to 88% in 2017. However, in Estonia, the percentage of patients who had a consultation with a specialist within 6 weeks was at 78% in 2013-15, then dropped to 73% in 2017 and again to 68% in 2018 (Figure 4.27).

Figure 4.27. Some Nordic countries have achieved progress in the percentage of persons meeting mental health waiting times target set in each country

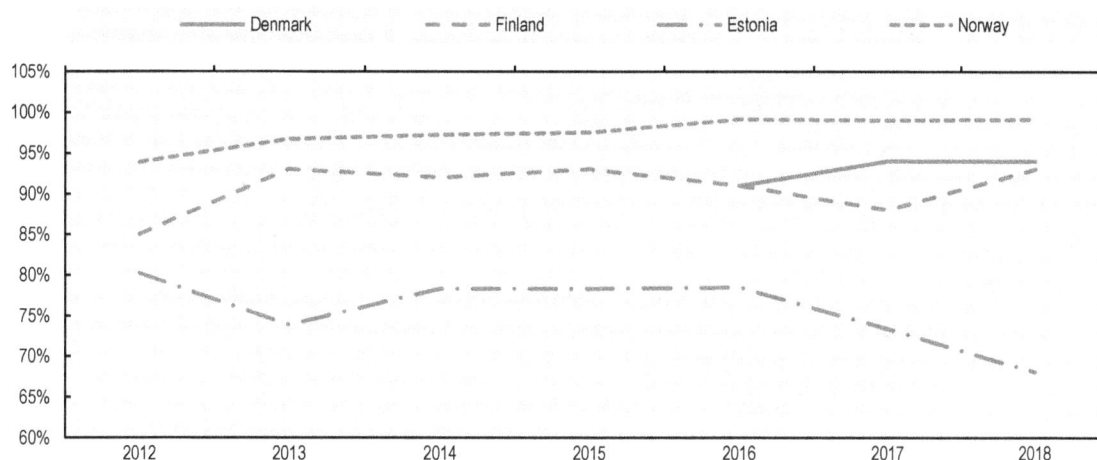

Note: Data show the percentage of persons who meet nationally-set wait times target for mental health services. The data are not comparable across countries because they cover different mental health services and waiting time targets for these services. National wait times shown are as follows: Denmark (persons assessed and investigated within 30 days); Finland (patients waiting less than 90 days before receiving psychiatric care following special assessment); Estonia (percentage of patients who had a consultation with a specialist within 6 weeks); Norway (percentage of patients who have received health care within the clinically assessed deadline assigned to the patient);.
Source: OECD Waiting Times Data Questionnaire 2019.

When looking at a broader measure of the average waiting times for all patients, there also appears to have been progress in reducing waiting times in these countries. Mean wait from referral to the start of treatment fell from 35 days in 2014 to 21 days in 2018 in Denmark; and from 52 days in 2014 to 45 days in 2018 in Norway. In Norway, average waiting time for adults fell by 2 days between 2018 and 2019, and 11 days between 2013 and 2019 (Helsedirektoratets Norway, 2019[48]). On the other hand, the mean waiting time to get a consultation with a mental health specialist rose slightly from 28 days in 2015 to 31 days in 2018 in Poland.

National aggregates can also mask variations by age group and region. For example in New Zealand, 91% of people under 19, 94% of working age adults (19 – 64) and 96% of older adults were seen by a mental health provider in under 8 weeks, a national total of 93% in 2017-18 (National Services Framework Library, 2019[49]). While in most regions more than 90% of people were seen by mental health services in less than 8 weeks, in the Southern region 87% of people had been seen. Another outlier stood out in the Taranaki region, where 23% of under 19 years olds waited longer than 8 weeks in 2017-18, more than twice the national average of 9%. However, it is not clear based on this analysis whether tracking wait times or introducing wait time targets in itself contributes to stabilised or falling average waits for mental health services. It may be that wait time tracking or targets are introduced in priority areas where other policy measures or investments are contributing to improving overall access.

It is important to pay attention not just to the proportion of people who were able to access care within a set waiting time target, but also to the range of wait times for services. For example, a majority of people may receive care within a certain number of weeks, but if a small number of people are still waiting two or three times longer to access care, this can point to areas of weakness in service provision.

4.4.5. Supply-side policies appear to be the most common tool for reducing mental health waiting times

Although policy discussions are not always framed in terms of reducing mental health wait times, or meeting maximum wait time targets, policies appear to be focused on better meeting demand through increased service volumes or scope, rather than managing demand. A primary driver for waiting times targets is to increase overall access to mental health services, linked to a broader recognition that a significant treatment gap exists in the area of mental health (OECD, 2014[50]; OECD/European Union, 2018[40]). Countries also identify shorter wait times for accessing services as a way to reduce the risk of deterioration in health, and improve outcomes from treatment (Helsedirektoratets Norway, 2019[48]; NHS England, 2015[43]).

For example, when England introduced maximum wait time targets for mental health services, this included an injection of funding of GBP 80 million to increase service capacity. This included GBP 40 million of recurrent funding to support increased capacity in order to meet the 2 week wait time target for early access to psychosis services. GBP 10 million was provided as implementation funding for psychological therapies services, which was to be used to confirm the accuracy of existing waiting lists, and enhance capacity to provide assessment and treatment (NHS England, 2015[43]).

In Australia, the 2019-20 health budget includes a priority focus on mental health. As part of this budget the Government will expand the 'headspace' service network, which provides care for young people, to improve access to services and reduce wait for services. A previous report had detailed that youth mental health services were coming under increasing demand for services, and that waiting times were a concern in almost 90% of youth mental health 'headspace' centres (headspace, 2019[51]). Under the 2019-20 budget, AUD 111.3 million (about USD 76 million) will be invested by 2021 to introduce 30 new centres or satellite centres, and AUD 152 million to help headspace centres experiencing high levels of demand (Australian Government Department of Health, 2019[52]). Waiting times will be tracked in headspace centres, which will be a tool to assess responsiveness to demand as well as the impact of additional funding.

In countries where waiting times are common across health services, introducing waiting times for mental health services can be part of a broader drive to create 'parity of esteem' between mental health care and the rest of the health care system, for example in England (NHS, 2019[53]). In Sweden and Denmark it appears that maximum waiting times targets for mental health are set to the same level as wait times for specialist services more broadly.

Based on information reported to the OECD, only Denmark has built in 'sanctions' in instances where maximum waiting time targets are not met. In Denmark extended free hospital choice means people have the right to receive examination or treatment in a private hospital if you have to wait more than 30 days.

5 Conclusion

Waiting times usually arise as the result of an imbalance between the demand for and the supply of health services. Although some waiting times can improve the efficiency of resources by reducing idle capacity, these efficiency gains are exhausted rapidly and when waiting times become long (e.g. above two or three months) patient dissatisfaction will increase. Addressing long waiting times for at least some health services was already a challenge for most OECD countries before the COVID-19 crisis, and the challenge will be exacerbated during and after the crisis as treatments and elective surgery are postponed. As a result policy makers will have to trigger changes to improve the appropriateness, responsiveness and efficiency in health service delivery. Such changes also provide an opportunity to make health systems more people centred by measuring waiting times along the patient pathway.

Waiting times for elective surgery, which are usually the longest, stalled in many countries over the past decade or increased at least slightly in others even before the COVID-19 crisis (e.g. Canada, Estonia, Ireland, Portugal). Denmark, England and Finland succeeded in reducing waiting times for many elective health services and maintained these reductions over sustained periods at least before the COVID-19 pandemic, although in some of these countries waiting times started to increase again as the demand for elective surgery grew faster than the supply.

The right policy mix to address long waiting times is likely to depend on the health system in each country. However, successful approaches typically combine the specification of an appropriate maximum waiting time together with supply-side and demand-side interventions and a regular monitoring of progress. Maximum waiting times can then be used as a target for the provider and/or a guarantee for the patient (as in England and Finland), with penalties for providers not meeting these targets. Waiting time guarantees can also be linked with patient choice policies (as in Denmark and Portugal), whereby patients are offered a greater choice of providers (including private hospitals) when they approach or reach the maximum waiting times without any additional cost for them. On the supply side, only permanent and sustained increases in supply can lead to permanent reductions in waiting times. The Netherlands is an example of a country that increased activity at a rapid pace in the 2000s through a range of supply initiatives that did reduce waiting times over that decade, though waiting times started to rise again in recent years even before the COVID-19 outbreak.

However, supply-side policies on their own are unlikely to deliver the expected reductions in waiting times. The main risk is that the additional supply is offset by an increase in demand, through an increase in referrals, tests and procedures, some of which may be inappropriate. Countries need to ensure that supply-side policies are linked to maximum waiting time enforcement to avoid disappointment. A demand-side approach is also necessary to rationalise either GP referrals to specialists, or the propensity of specialists to add patients to a waiting list. Maximum waiting times can act as an indirect policy lever to ensure that when supply increases providers do not offset these by increasing demand (though supply-induced demand or inappropriate referrals).

Policy makers can also introduce several complementary and more direct approaches on the demand side to reduce waiting times for elective treatment (as in New Zealand), though acknowledging any explicit reduction in demand can be politically challenging (as it can be interpreted as rationing access to care). Clinical prioritisation tools that distinguish between patients with different health benefits and severity can improve the referral process and the composition of the patients on the list. Prioritisation policies can also help to re-allocate waiting times by letting patients with more severe conditions wait less than those with less severe conditions (as in Norway). Strengthening the primary care referral systems from primary to second care, and improving the coordination between primary and secondary care, is a key policy to ensure the resources are used efficiently and to reduce waiting times.

The traditional focus has been on measuring and addressing waiting times in elective care, an area where measures of waiting times have improved by taking a broader look at the entire referral-to-treatment waiting time rather than focussing only on the last part of the patient journey after specialists have added patients to waiting lists. A growing number of OECD countries also measure waiting times in other areas, including in primary care, for hospital emergency department visits, mental health services or cancer care. Waiting times in primary care are less often considered a policy concern than in elective care, and only a few countries (such as Finland, Norway, and Spain) have implemented maximum waiting times to get an appointment with a general practitioner (family doctor) or other primary care providers. Policies in primary care often focus on increasing the supply of general practitioners, nurses and appointment slots. However, more and more countries (such as Australia, Luxembourg and Estonia) are exploiting the potential of new technologies (e.g. teleconsultations) to improve timely access to primary care, and the implementation of teleconsultations and other digital health tools have accelerated during the COVID-19 crisis.

More than half of OECD countries have developed waiting time strategies for cancer care covering both diagnosis and treatment, sometimes as part of national cancer control plans. Countries, such as Denmark, Ireland, Latvia, Poland, Slovenia and Spain, have also introduced fast track pathways for cancer patients, sometimes facilitated by additional dedicated funding and capacity and efforts to improve coordination.

Policies to reduce waiting times policies for mental health services appear to be focused on better meeting demand through increased service volume or scope, rather than managing demand, possibly due to historical underfunding of mental health. In some cases, waiting time targets are part of a drive to increase overall access to mental health services, linked to a broader recognition that a significant treatment gap exists in this clinical area.

References

Abásolo, I., M. Negrín-Hernández and J. Pinilla (2014), "Equity in specialist waiting times by socioeconomic groups: Evidence from Spain", *European Journal of Health Economics*, Vol. 15/3, pp. 323-334, http://dx.doi.org/10.1007/s10198-013-0524-x.   [16]

Australian Government Department of Health (2019), *Prioritising Mental Health – national headspace network*.   [52]

Bird, V. et al. (2010), *Early intervention services, cognitive-behavioural therapy and family intervention in early psychosis: Systematic review*, http://dx.doi.org/10.1192/bjp.bp.109.074526.   [22]

Biringer, E. et al. (2015), "Life on a waiting list: How do people experience and cope with delayed access to a community mental health center?", *Scandinavian Psychologist*, Vol. 2, http://dx.doi.org/10.15714/scandpsychol.2.e6.   [31]

Canadian Psychiatric Association (2006), *Wait Time Benchmarks for Patients With Serious Psychiatric Illnesses*.   [42]

Children's Mental Health Ontario (2020), *Kids Can't Wait: 2020 Report on Wait Lists and Wait Times for Child and Youth Mental Health Care in Ontario*, Children's Mental Health Ontario, https://www.cmho.org/images/policy-papers/CMHO-Report-WaitTimes-2020.pdf (accessed on 30 March 2020).   [47]

CIHI (2019), *Wait times for joint replacements and cataract surgery growing in much of Canada | CIHI*, https://www.cihi.ca/en/wait-times-for-joint-replacements-and-cataract-surgery-growing-in-much-of-canada (accessed on 20 November 2019).   [33]

Global News Canada (2020), "Ontario child and youth mental health service wait lists double: Report", https://globalnews.ca/news/6467545/ontario-youth-mental-health-wait-list/ (accessed on 30 March 2020).   [45]

Government Inquiry into Mental Health and Addiction (2018), *He Ara Oranga : Report of the Government Inquiry into Mental Health and Addiction*, https://mentalhealth.inquiry.govt.nz/inquiry-report/he-ara-oranga/chapter-2-what-we-heard-the-voices-of-the-people/2-10-access-wait-times-and-quality/ (accessed on 25 October 2019).   [30]

Gravelle, H. and L. Siciliani (2008), "Ramsey waits: Allocating public health service resources when there is rationing by waiting", *Journal of Health Economics*, Vol. 27/5, pp. 1143-1154, http://dx.doi.org/10.1016/j.jhealeco.2008.03.004.   [6]

headspace (2019), *Increasing demand in youth mental health: A rising tide of need.* [51]

Helsedirektoratets Norway (2019), *Shorter waiting time in mental health care and intoxication treatment*, [48]
https://translate.google.com/translate?hl=fr&sl=auto&tl=en&u=https%3A%2F%2Fwww.regjeri
ngen.no%2Fno%2Faktuelt%2Fkortere-ventetid-innen-psykisk-helsevern-og-
rusbehandling%2Fid2662205%2F (accessed on 25 October 2019).

Hurst, J. and L. Siciliani (2003), "Tackling Excessive Waiting Times for Elective Surgery: A Comparison of Policies in Twelve OECD Countries", *OECD Health Working Papers*, No. 6, OECD Publishing, Paris, https://dx.doi.org/10.1787/108471127058. [32]

Ipsos (2020), *Children's Mental Health Ontario*, https://www.ipsos.com/en-ca/news-polls/28000- [46]
Children-And-Youth-On-Wait-Lists-For-Mental-Health-Services-In-Ontario (accessed on
30 March 2020).

Johar, M. et al. (2013), "Discrimination in a universal health system: Explaining socioeconomic waiting time gaps", *Journal of Health Economics*, Vol. 32/1, pp. 181-194, http://dx.doi.org/10.1016/j.jhealeco.2012.09.004. [7]

Kaarboe, O. and F. Carlsen (2014), "Waiting times and socioeconomic status. Evidence from Norway", *Health Economics (United Kingdom)*, Vol. 23/1, pp. 93-107, http://dx.doi.org/10.1002/hec.2904. [12]

Kowalewski, K., J. McLennan and P. McGrath (2011), "A preliminary investigation of wait times for child and adolescent mental health services in Canada", *Journal of the Canadian Academy of Child and Adolescent Psychiatry*, Vol. 20/2, pp. 112-119. [26]

Landi, S., E. Ivaldi and A. Testi (2018), *Socioeconomic status and waiting times for health services: An international literature review and evidence from the Italian National Health System*, Elsevier Ireland Ltd, http://dx.doi.org/10.1016/j.healthpol.2018.01.003. [17]

Laudicella, M., L. Siciliani and R. Cookson (2012), "Waiting times and socioeconomic status: Evidence from England", *Social Science and Medicine*, Vol. 74/9, pp. 1331-1341, http://dx.doi.org/10.1016/j.socscimed.2011.12.049. [9]

Ministry of Health, Labour and Welfare (2019), *Heisei 29nen Juryou Koudou Chosa (kakuteisuu) no Gaikyo*, https://www.mhlw.go.jp/toukei/saikin/hw/jyuryo/17/kakutei.html (accessed on 20 November 2019). [54]

Monstad, K., L. Engesaeter and B. Espehaug (2014), "Waiting time and socioeconomic status - An individual-level analysis", *Health Economics*, Vol. 23/4, pp. 446-461, http://dx.doi.org/10.1002/hec.2924. [11]

Moscelli, G. et al. (2018), "Socioeconomic inequality of access to healthcare: Does choice explain the gradient?", *Journal of Health Economics*, Vol. 57, pp. 290-314, http://dx.doi.org/10.1016/j.jhealeco.2017.06.005. [10]

Moscelli, G., L. Siciliani and V. Tonei (2016), *Do waiting times affect health outcomes? Evidence from coronary bypass*, Elsevier Ltd, http://dx.doi.org/10.1016/j.socscimed.2016.05.043. [20]

National Services Framework Library (2019), *PP8: Shorter waits for non-urgent mental health and addiction services, see mental health and addictions waiting time data*, https://nsfl.health.govt.nz/accountability/performance-and-monitoring/mental-health-alcohol-and-drug-addiction-sector (accessed on 25 October 2019). [49]

Nederlandse Zorgautoriteit (2018), *Wachttijden in de gespecialiseerde ggz (Waiting times in specialist mental healthcare)*, https://www.staatvenz.nl/kerncijfers/wachttijden-de-gespecialiseerde-ggz (accessed on 27 March 2020). [41]

NHS (2019), *Investment and evolution: A five-year framework for GP contract reform to implement The NHS Long Term Plan*. [36]

NHS (2019), *The NHS Long Term Plan*, http://www.longtermplan.nhs.uk (accessed on 25 October 2019). [53]

NHS England (2015), *Guidance to support the introduction of access and waiting time standards for mental health services in 2015/16*. [43]

NICE (2014), *Costing statement: Psychosis and schizophrenia in adults: treatment and management Implementing the NICE guideline on Psychosis and schizophrenia in adults (CG178) Putting NICE guidance into practice*. [44]

Nikolova, S., M. Harrison and M. Sutton (2016), "The Impact of Waiting Time on Health Gains from Surgery: Evidence from a National Patient-reported Outcome Dataset", *Health Economics (United Kingdom)*, Vol. 25/8, pp. 955-968, http://dx.doi.org/10.1002/hec.3195. [21]

OECD (2020), "Beyond containment: Health systems responses to COVID-19 in the OECD", *OECD Policy Responses to Coronavirus (Covid-19)*, http://www.oecd.org/coronavirus/policy-responses/beyond-containment-health-systems-responses-to-covid-19-in-the-oecd-6ab740c0/. [34]

OECD (2020), *Realising the Potential of Primary Health Care*, OECD Health Policy Studies, OECD Publishing, Paris, https://dx.doi.org/10.1787/a92adee4-en. [35]

OECD (2019), *Health for Everyone?: Social Inequalities in Health and Health Systems*, OECD Health Policy Studies, OECD Publishing, Paris, https://dx.doi.org/10.1787/3c8385d0-en. [55]

OECD (2017), *Tackling Wasteful Spending on Health*, OECD Publishing, Paris, https://dx.doi.org/10.1787/9789264266414-en. [5]

OECD (2016), *Health System Characteristics Survey*, http://www.oecd.org/els/health-systems/characteristics.htm. [37]

OECD (2014), *Geographic Variations in Health Care: What Do We Know and What Can Be Done to Improve Health System Performance?*, OECD Health Policy Studies, OECD Publishing, Paris, https://dx.doi.org/10.1787/9789264216594-en. [4]

OECD (2014), *Making Mental Health Count: The Social and Economic Costs of Neglecting Mental Health Care*, OECD Health Policy Studies, OECD Publishing, Paris, https://dx.doi.org/10.1787/9789264208445-en. [50]

OECD (2013), *Cancer Care: Assuring Quality to Improve Survival*, OECD Health Policy Studies, OECD Publishing, Paris, https://dx.doi.org/10.1787/9789264181052-en. [39]

OECD (2012), *Sick on the Job?: Myths and Realities about Mental Health and Work*, Mental Health and Work, OECD Publishing, Paris, https://dx.doi.org/10.1787/9789264124523-en. [28]

OECD/European Union (2018), *Health at a Glance: Europe 2018: State of Health in the EU Cycle*, OECD Publishing, Paris/European Union, Brussels, https://dx.doi.org/10.1787/health_glance_eur-2018-en. [40]

Oliveira Hashiguchi, T. (2020), "Bringing health care to the patient: An overview of the use of telemedicine in OECD countries", *OECD Health Working Papers*, No. 116, OECD Publishing, Paris, https://dx.doi.org/10.1787/8e56ede7-en. [38]

Reichert, A. and R. Jacobs (2018), "The impact of waiting time on patient outcomes: Evidence from early intervention in psychosis services in England", *Health Economics (United Kingdom)*, Vol. 27/11, pp. 1772-1787, http://dx.doi.org/10.1002/hec.3800. [23]

Royal College of Psychiatrists (2018), *Long waits for mental health treatment lead to divorce, job loss and money problems, RCPsych finds*, https://www.rcpsych.ac.uk/news-and-features/latest-news/detail/2018/10/08/long-waits-for-mental-health-treatment-lead-to-divorce-job-loss-and-money-problems-rcpsych-finds (accessed on 28 October 2019). [29]

Schraeder, K. and G. Reid (2015), "Why Wait? The Effect of Wait-Times on Subsequent Help-Seeking Among Families Looking for Children's Mental Health Services", *Journal of Abnormal Child Psychology*, Vol. 43/3, pp. 553-565, http://dx.doi.org/10.1007/s10802-014-9928-z. [24]

Sharma, A., L. Siciliani and A. Harris (2013), "Waiting times and socioeconomic status: Does sample selection matter?", *Economic Modelling*, Vol. 33, pp. 659-667, http://dx.doi.org/10.1016/j.econmod.2013.05.009. [8]

Siciliani, L. (2015), "Waiting Times: Evidence of Social Inequalities in Access for Care", in *Data and Measures in Health Services Research*, Springer US, http://dx.doi.org/10.1007/978-1-4899-7673-4_17-1. [2]

Siciliani, L., M. Borowitz and V. Moran (eds.) (2013), *Waiting Time Policies in the Health Sector: What Works?*, OECD Health Policy Studies, OECD Publishing, Paris, https://dx.doi.org/10.1787/9789264179080-en. [1]

Siciliani, L. and R. Verzulli (2009), "Waiting times and socioeconomic status among elderly europeans: Evidence from share", *Health Economics*, Vol. 18/11, pp. 1295-1306, http://dx.doi.org/10.1002/hec.1429. [15]

Smirthwaite, G. et al. (2016), "Inequity in waiting for cataract surgery - An analysis of data from the Swedish National Cataract Register", *International Journal for Equity in Health*, Vol. 15/1, http://dx.doi.org/10.1186/s12939-016-0302-3. [14]

Sobolev, B. and G. Fradet (2008), "Delays for coronary artery bypass surgery: How long is too long?", *Expert Review of Pharmacoeconomics and Outcomes Research*, Vol. 8/1, pp. 27-32, http://dx.doi.org/10.1586/14737167.8.1.27. [18]

Sobolev, B. et al. (2012), "An observational study to evaluate 2 target times for elective coronary bypass surgery", *Medical Care*, Vol. 50/7, pp. 611-619, http://dx.doi.org/10.1097/MLR.0b013e31824deed2. [19]

Tinghög, G. et al. (2014), "Horizontal inequality in rationing by waiting lists", *International Journal of Health Services*, Vol. 44/1, pp. 169-184, http://dx.doi.org/10.2190/HS.44.1.j.   [13]

Wennberg, J. (2010), *Tracking Medicine: A Researcher's Quest to Understand Health Care*, Oxford University Press (OUP).   [3]

Westin, A., C. Barksdale and S. Stephan (2014), "The effect of waiting time on youth engagement to evidence based treatments", *Community Mental Health Journal*, Vol. 50/2, pp. 221-228, http://dx.doi.org/10.1007/s10597-012-9585-z.   [25]

Williams, M., J. Latta and P. Conversano (2008), "Eliminating the wait for mental health services", *Journal of Behavioral Health Services and Research*, Vol. 35/1, pp. 107-114, http://dx.doi.org/10.1007/s11414-007-9091-1.   [27]

Annex A. Identifying good practices to measure waiting times

The measurement of waiting times varies widely across OECD countries, from no measurement in countries where this is not perceived to be an important policy issue to sophisticated and comprehensive measurement in some countries where this is considered to be a high priority. This annex provides an overview of different measures of waiting times and identifies good practices.

The two most common measures are waiting times of patients treated and waiting times of patients on the list

An important aspect in measurement relates to the distinction between two distributions of waiting times: i) the distribution of waiting times of *patients treated* in a given period (for example, a financial year, a quarter or a month); ii) the distribution of waiting times of the *patients still on the list* at a point in time (a census date, e.g. first Monday of the month or 31st of December). The first distribution measures the full duration of the patient's waiting time experience (from entering to exiting the list). The second distribution relates to an "incomplete" waiting time measure since the patient's wait has yet to come to an end (they are still on the list).

The waiting time of patients treated has the advantage of capturing the full duration of a patient's journey, but is retrospective in nature. The main advantage of the waiting time of patients on the list is that it captures the experience of the patients who are still waiting at a point in time and can give 'live' updates. However, the distribution of the waiting time of the patient on the list oversamples patients with long waiting times, while patients with short duration disappear more quickly from the list. As a result, the mean or median waiting time of patients on the list is not necessarily lower than the waiting time of patients treated, as one may intuitively expect.

Another difference between the two distributions is that the wait on the list includes not only patients who will receive treatment at some point in the future but also those who will not, namely patients who give up the treatment while waiting, die or receive treatment by another provider. These may increase the waiting time of the patients on the list if the waiting list records are not updated regularly.

England is one country that reports both the waiting time of the patients on the list and the waiting time of the patients treated, where waiting time is based on a comprehensive referral-to-treatment (RTT) approach that distinguishes patients who were admitted to hospital from those who were not admitted. The following table covers the twelve-months period from August 2018 and July 2019 and illustrates how the median waiting time can differ across measures.

Table A A.1. Referral to Treatment (RTT) Waiting Times, England

Month	Incomplete RTT pathways	Admitted RTT pathways	Non-Admitted RTT pathways
	Median wait (weeks)	Median wait (weeks)	Median wait (weeks)
Aug-18	7.5	9.7	5.8
Sep-18	7.6	10.4	6.5
Oct-18	7.0	10.4	6.1
Nov-18	6.9	10.0	6.0
Dec-18	7.6	9.2	5.6
Jan-19	7.8	10.7	6.7
Feb-19	6.7	10.8	5.8
Mar-19	6.9	10.3	5.6
Apr-19	7.2	10.0	5.8
May-19	7.7	10.3	6.3
Jun-19	7.5	10.6	6.2
Jul-19	7.3	10.2	6.1
Aug-18	7.5	9.7	5.8
Sep-18	7.6	10.4	6.5

Source: NHS England and NHS Improvement: monthly RTT data collection https://www.england.nhs.uk/statistics/statistical-work-areas/rtt-waiting-times/rtt-data-2019-20/.

Comprehensive measures of waiting times are more informative than more partial measures

There are different possible start and end points to waiting times, as shown in Table A A.1 above. The waiting time can be recorded from the GP referral or following a specialist visit. It can end with a surgery or medical treatment, or with a specialist visit. Some health systems measure what is sometimes referred to as the "outpatient" waiting time (from GP referral to specialist visit), others the "inpatient" waiting time (from specialist decision to add the patient on the list to treatment), yet others measure the overall referral-to-treatment waiting time (from GP referral to treatment), as is the case in Denmark, Norway and England.[7]

Capturing the distribution of waiting times of patients treated or on the list

The most common statistics to measure the waiting times of patients treated or on the list are: the mean waiting time, the median waiting time or the waiting time at other percentiles of the distribution, for example the 75th, or 95th percentile. Many countries also report the number or proportion of patients waiting more than a threshold waiting time (for example 3, 6 or 12 months).

The distribution of waiting times is generally skewed, with a small proportion of patients waiting a very long time. Hence, the mean can be substantially longer than the median. Although the mean and median are representative of the average patient's experience, measures that focus on the tail of the distribution help to identify those patients whose wait is longest, though as long as prioritisation works well, these patients are also likely to be patients with the lowest need or severity.

Administrative databases can provide more specific and regular data, but population-based surveys can also provide some useful additional information from the patient perspective

Most information on waiting times is available from administrative databases in countries where waiting times are considered to be a significant policy issue. Survey data is also available for a subset of countries (e.g. Australia, as well as other countries participating in the Commonwealth Fund International Health Policy Survey). While administrative databases can provide more regular and reliable data on waiting times for specific health services by region and by setting (e.g. at the hospital or general practice level), surveys can also provide useful complementary information as experienced by patients and some indication of possible inequalities in waiting times by gender, age and socioeconomic status (e.g. by income level), particularly if the sample size is large enough (though in some countries, in particular the Nordic countries, this is also possible with administrative data).

Notes

[1] Japan conducts a survey on patient experience every three years, including questions on waiting times. The results for the last wave conducted in 2017 show that the waiting time between the time when a doctor referred a patient for inpatient care and the time when the hospitalisation occurred was within one week for 56% of patients while the proportion who waited more than one month was 13%. The main reasons for waits of over more one month was the limited availability of resources such as beds, diagnostic tests and surgeries (34%) and personal and/or other family circumstances (23%) (Ministry of Health, Labour and Welfare, 2019[54]).

[2] Results from another European-wide survey carried out in 2014 (the European Health Interview Survey, EHIS) show greater levels of people reporting delay in getting an appointment for health care due to waiting times, ranging from about 4% of respondents in Norway to about 30% in Luxembourg. Part of the reason for these higher rates are that these survey results exclude those people who didn't have any health care needs (OECD, 2019[55]).

[3] The study on coronary bypass by Moscelli et al. (2018[10]) also shows that inequalities are more pronounced when waiting times are long (e.g. above 150 days) but reduce proportionally (or more than proportionally) when waiting times reduce to shorter levels (60 days on average). This suggests that when waiting times are shorter, individuals with higher socio-economic status feel less pressured to identify mechanisms to avoid waiting.

[4] In April 2019, patients had been waiting for elective care in hospitals for approximately 1-2 months, with those waiting between 3 and 6 months accounting for 13% of all patients. However, their number has increased from the previous year (by 1 400 people).

[5] It may be assumed that where not otherwise specified, these waiting times are for non-urgent cases.

[6] In its response to the OECD Policy questionnaire in September 2019, the Slovak Republic also indicated that it was in the process of drafting a legislation on maximum waiting times for specific treatments, including possibly for mental health services, while Poland tracks waiting times data.

[7] Along the pathway patients may need a diagnostic test (e.g. an MRI or CT scan). Therefore, some health systems may record the waiting time from GP referral to a diagnostic test or from specialist request to diagnostic test, and this may or may not be included in the inpatient waiting time.

www.ingramcontent.com/pod-product-compliance
Lightning Source LLC
Chambersburg PA
CBHW080340270326
41927CB00014B/3301